NO SUGAR-DIET FOR BEGINNERS

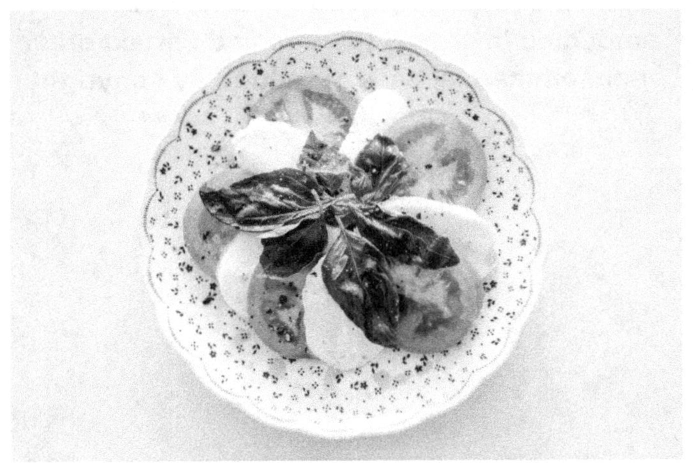

Transform Your Health Through Sugar-Free Recipes, Weight Loss Strategies, Diabetes Management, and Lower Cholesterol

Thelma Howard

Table of Contents

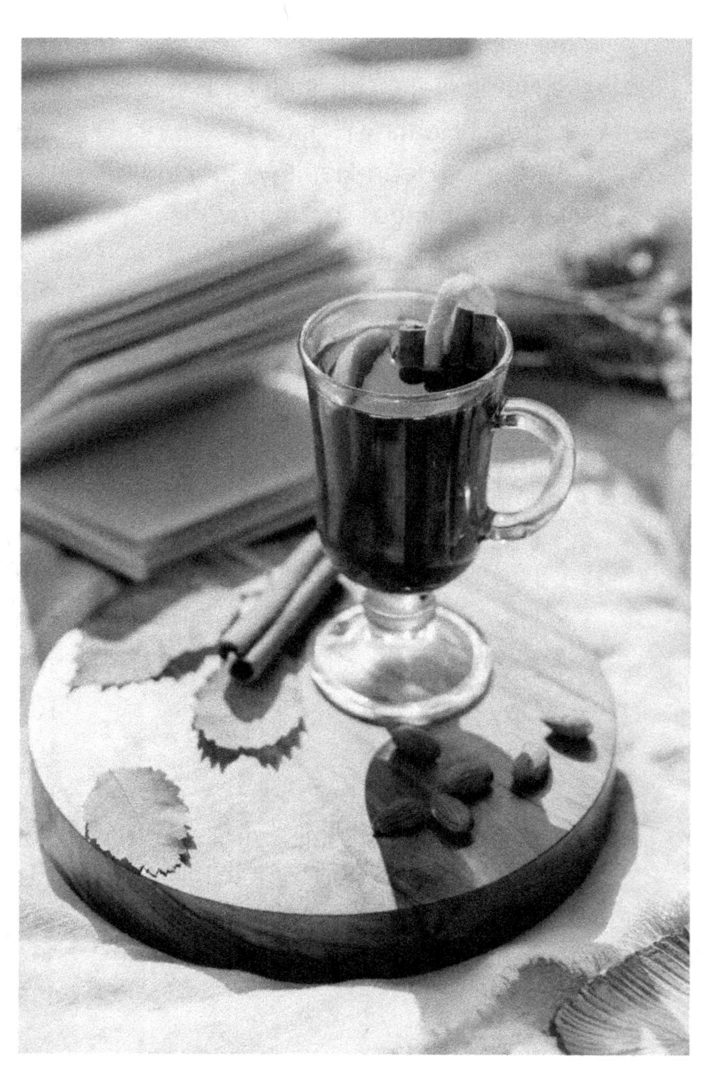

INTRODUCTION

In a world saturated with sugary temptations, Thelma found herself at a crossroads, grappling with the repercussions of her sugar-laden lifestyle. Fueled by a desire for change, she embarked on a transformative journey toward a healthier, sugar-free existence. As her body adapted to a newfound vitality, Thelma became inspired to share her experience with others.

Enter "No Sugar Diet for Beginners," a comprehensive guide that serves as a roadmap for those seeking a life free from the shackles of excessive sugar consumption. This book is more than just a collection of recipes; it's a holistic approach to well-being, encompassing weight loss strategies, diabetes management, and cholesterol reduction.

Readers are invited to explore the delicious realm of sugar-free recipes that not only nourish the body but also tantalize the taste buds. The pages unfold with practical tips, empowering individuals to make informed choices and break free from the addictive cycle of sugar.
As the narrative unfolds, readers will discover that the journey to optimal health is not only attainable but also enjoyable. With "No Sugar Diet for Beginners," embark on a path to transformation, where vibrant health and well-being become the sweetest rewards.

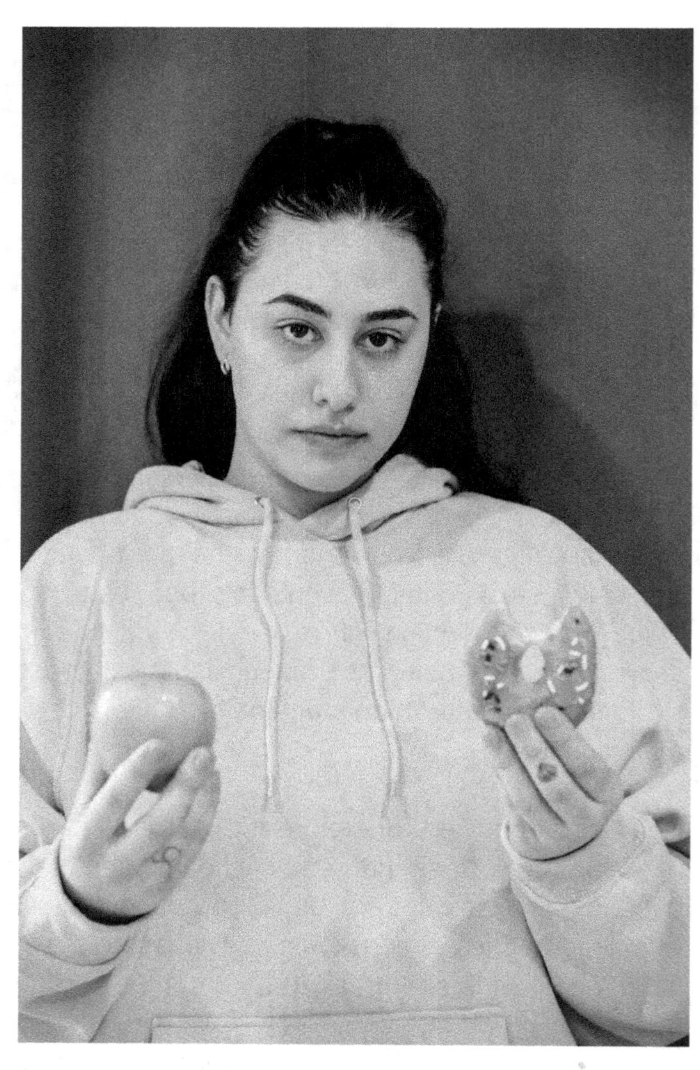

CHAPTER ONE

Understanding the Impact of Sugar on Health

The introduction to a sugar-free lifestyle begins with a profound understanding of how sugar influences our health. This section delves into the various ways excessive sugar consumption affects the body, from immediate physiological responses to long-term health implications.

Blood Sugar Spikes and Crashes

Our bodies need blood sugar, often known as glucose, as a source of energy. However, the consumption of sugary foods can lead to a rollercoaster effect, characterized by rapid spikes and subsequent crashes in blood sugar levels. Understanding the dynamics of blood sugar spikes and crashes empowers individuals to make informed dietary choices, promoting stable energy levels and overall well-being. It forms a crucial aspect of adopting a sugar-free lifestyle for enhanced health and vitality.

1. **Sugar Spike Mechanism**

When we consume foods high in refined sugars, the body quickly converts them into glucose, causing a sudden surge in blood sugar levels. This spike triggers the release of insulin from the pancreas to help cells absorb and utilize the excess glucose for energy.

2. Energetic Highs and Lows

During the initial phase of elevated blood sugar, individuals may experience a burst of energy and heightened alertness. This temporary surge is often followed by a rapid decline, leaving individuals feeling fatigued, irritable, and craving more sugary snacks to regain energy.

3. Consequences of Blood Sugar Crashes

The abrupt drop in blood sugar can lead to symptoms like shakiness, weakness, dizziness, and difficulty concentrating. The body perceives this as a state of emergency, prompting further cravings for quick sources of energy, often leading to a cycle of overeating and poor food choices.

4. Impact on Weight Management

Frequent blood sugar spikes and crashes disrupt the body's ability to regulate appetite, making it challenging to maintain a healthy weight. Unstable blood sugar levels contribute to overeating and cravings for high-calorie, sugary foods.

5. Long-Term Health Implications

Chronic exposure to this cycle is associated with an increased risk of insulin resistance, a precursor to type 2 diabetes. Prolonged insulin resistance can contribute to weight gain, inflammation, and various metabolic disorders.

6. **Strategies for Blood Sugar Stability**
Choosing complex carbohydrates and fiber-rich foods to promote gradual glucose release. Balancing meals with a combination of proteins, healthy fats, and carbohydrates to provide sustained energy. Monitoring and managing portion sizes to prevent excessive glucose influx.

Weight Gain and Obesity

The global surge in weight gain and obesity is intricately tied to dietary habits, with excessive sugar consumption playing a pivotal role in this alarming trend.Understanding the intricate relationship between excessive sugar consumption and weight gain is a vital step toward breaking the cycle of obesity. By making informed dietary choices, individuals can pave the way for sustainable weight management and improved health.

Understanding how sugar contributes to weight gain and obesity is crucial for those seeking a healthier lifestyle.

1. **Caloric Overload**
Sugary foods and beverages are often calorie-dense, contributing to an imbalance between energy intake and expenditure. The excess calories, especially when derived from

added sugars, are stored in the body as fat, leading to weight gain over time.

2. Insulin Resistance and Fat Storage

High sugar intake prompts the pancreas to release insulin to manage the increased glucose levels. Prolonged exposure to elevated insulin levels can lead to insulin resistance, causing the body to store more fat, particularly around the abdomen.

3. Leptin Resistance

Leptin is a hormone that regulates hunger and signals feelings of fullness. Excessive sugar consumption can lead to leptin resistance, disrupting the body's ability to recognize when it is full, potentially resulting in overeating.

4. Inflammation and Fat Deposition

High sugar intake triggers inflammation, promoting the storage of fat cells. Chronic inflammation is associated with the development of obesity and related metabolic disorders.

5. Craving Cycle and Emotional Eating

Sugary foods can create a cycle of cravings, leading to frequent snacking and overconsumption. Emotional eating, often triggered by stress or mood fluctuations, can further contribute to unhealthy weight gain.

6. **Metabolic Syndrome and Increased Risks**

Obesity is a key component of metabolic syndrome, a cluster of conditions that elevate the risk of heart disease, diabetes, and stroke. Excess sugar intake is linked to the development of metabolic syndrome, amplifying the health risks associated with obesity.

7. **Strategies for Weight Management**

Adopting a balanced diet rich in whole foods, emphasizing fruits, vegetables, lean proteins, and whole grains. Reducing or eliminating added sugars and processed foods to create a calorie deficit.

- Incorporating regular physical activity to support weight loss and overall well-being.

Inflammation and Chronic Diseases

Inflammation, typically the body's defense mechanism against harm, can become a silent assailant when chronic and triggered by a high intake of added sugars. This connection between inflammation and excessive sugar consumption has far-reaching implications for the development and progression of chronic diseases. Understanding the intricate link between excessive sugar intake and chronic inflammation underscores the importance of dietary choices in preventing and managing a spectrum of chronic diseases. By adopting an anti-inflammatory lifestyle, individuals can cultivate a foundation for long-term health and well-being.

1. **Inflammatory Response to Sugar**

The consumption of refined sugars stimulates the release of inflammatory messengers, such as cytokines, within the body. Chronic exposure to these inflammatory signals can lead to sustained low-grade inflammation, even in the absence of apparent injury or infection.

2. **Contribution to Chronic Diseases**

Prolonged inflammation is a common denominator in the development of various chronic diseases, including cardiovascular disease, diabetes, and certain cancers. The inflammatory process can exacerbate existing health conditions and contribute to their progression.

3. **Insulin Resistance and Inflammation**

Excessive sugar intake is closely linked to insulin resistance, a condition where cells become less responsive to insulin's signals. Insulin resistance not only disrupts glucose regulation but also fosters inflammation, creating a detrimental cycle.

4. **Impact on Cardiovascular Health**

Chronic inflammation is a key factor in atherosclerosis, the buildup of plaque in arteries that can lead to heart attacks and strokes. High sugar intake contributes to both inflammation and other cardiovascular risk factors, such as elevated blood pressure and cholesterol levels.

5. Connection to Autoimmune Disorders

Chronic inflammation may trigger or exacerbate autoimmune diseases, where the immune system mistakenly attacks the body's own tissues. Sugar-induced inflammation can amplify the severity of autoimmune conditions.

6. Joint Health and Inflammation

Inflammatory processes fueled by excessive sugar intake may contribute to joint pain and conditions like rheumatoid arthritis. Adopting an anti-inflammatory diet can alleviate symptoms and promote joint health.

7. Reducing Inflammation through Dietary Changes

Emphasizing a diet rich in anti-inflammatory foods, including fruits, vegetables, nuts, and fatty fish. Limiting the intake of added sugars, refined carbohydrates, and processed foods to mitigate inflammatory responses.

8. Lifestyle Factors and Inflammation

Regular physical activity, sufficient sleep, and stress management play pivotal roles in modulating inflammation. A holistic approach that addresses lifestyle factors can contribute to reducing chronic inflammation and mitigating associated health risks.

Impact on Mental Health

The influence of sugar on mental health extends beyond its impact on physical well-being, weaving a complex tapestry that involves neurotransmitters, mood regulation, and even the risk of mental health disorders. Recognizing the intricate interplay between sugar consumption and mental health empowers individuals to make mindful dietary choices that not only nourish the body but also nurture mental well-being. As part of a holistic approach to health, reducing sugar intake can contribute to a more stable and resilient mind. Understanding this connection is crucial for those seeking to nurture not just their bodies but also their mental resilience.

1. Neurotransmitter Disruption

Excessive sugar intake can disrupt the balance of neurotransmitters, such as serotonin and dopamine, which play key roles in regulating mood. Fluctuations in these neurotransmitters may contribute to symptoms of anxiety, depression, and mood swings.

2. Blood Sugar Fluctuations and Mood

Rapid spikes and crashes in blood sugar levels, often induced by sugary foods, can impact mood stability. Sugar-induced hypoglycemia may lead to irritability, fatigue, and difficulty concentrating, affecting overall mental well-being.

3. **Addictive Nature of Sugar**

Sugar activates the brain's reward system, triggering the release of feel-good neurotransmitters. The repetitive cycle of sugar consumption and reward can lead to addictive behaviors, with potential implications for mental health.

4. **Inflammation and Mental Health**

Chronic inflammation, associated with high sugar intake, has been linked to an increased risk of mental health disorders. Inflammatory processes may contribute to conditions like depression and cognitive decline.

5. **Cognitive Function and Sugar**

High sugar consumption has been associated with cognitive impairment and a higher risk of developing conditions such as dementia and Alzheimer's disease. Insulin resistance, a consequence of excessive sugar intake, may impact brain function and cognitive abilities.

6. **Emotional Eating and Coping Mechanisms**

Sugar is often used as a coping mechanism for stress, anxiety, or emotional distress. Addressing emotional eating habits is crucial for establishing healthier coping mechanisms and supporting mental resilience.

7. **Gut-Brain Connection**
According to new research, there is a direct link between the gut and the brain, and mental health is influenced by the gut flora. Excessive sugar consumption can negatively impact gut health, potentially affecting mental well-being.

8. **Promoting Mental Health through Nutrition**
Adopting a balanced diet with nutrient-rich foods to support brain function and neurotransmitter synthesis. Incorporating omega-3 fatty acids, antioxidants, and other brain-boosting nutrients for mental resilience.

Effects on Skin Health

Beyond its well-known effects on internal health, excessive sugar consumption can significantly influence the appearance and health of your skin. Understanding the intricate relationship between sugar and skin health is essential for those seeking a radiant complexion and overall well-being. Understanding the impact of sugar on skin health serves as a motivator for adopting a sugar-conscious lifestyle. By making mindful dietary choices, individuals can promote not only internal health but also cultivate a vibrant and youthful complexion.

1. **Formation of Advanced Glycation End Products (AGEs)**
Excess sugar in the bloodstream can lead to the formation of AGEs, compounds that damage proteins, including collagen and elastin crucial for skin elasticity. AGEs contribute to premature aging, leading to wrinkles, fine lines, and sagging skin.

2. **Inflammation and Acne Formation**
High sugar intake promotes inflammation, which can exacerbate skin conditions like acne. Inflammatory responses may trigger an overproduction of sebum, contributing to clogged pores and acne development.

3. **Collagen Breakdown**
Sugar disrupts the structure of collagen fibers, the building blocks of healthy skin. Collagen breakdown leads to decreased skin firmness and resilience, contributing to the appearance of aging.

4. **Skin Dehydration**
Sugary foods can contribute to dehydration, negatively impacting skin hydration levels. Dehydrated skin is more prone to dullness, flakiness, and an uneven complexion.

5. **Promotion of Glycation and Wrinkles**
Glycation, a process accelerated by sugar, involves the binding of sugar molecules to proteins like collagen. This process contributes to the formation

of wrinkles and the loss of skin's natural youthful appearance.

6. Impact on Skin Conditions
Sugar may exacerbate existing skin conditions such as eczema and psoriasis due to its inflammatory effects. Managing sugar intake can play a role in minimizing symptoms and promoting healthier skin.

7. Antioxidant Depletion
Excessive sugar consumption can deplete antioxidant levels in the body. Antioxidants are crucial for protecting the skin from oxidative stress and environmental damage.

8. Promoting a Skin-Friendly Diet
Embracing a diet rich in fruits, vegetables, and antioxidant-packed foods to support skin health. Hydrating adequately and choosing water over sugary beverages for optimal skin hydration.

Insulin Resistance and Type 2 Diabetes

The pervasive influence of excessive sugar consumption extends beyond immediate effects, playing a central role in the development of insulin resistance and, subsequently, type 2 diabetes. Understanding this intricate connection is vital for those navigating the complexities of metabolic health. Knowing the connection between excessive sugar consumption, insulin resistance, and type 2 diabetes empowers individuals to make informed lifestyle choices. By prioritizing a sugar-conscious approach to nutrition and embracing a health-conscious lifestyle, one can mitigate the risk factors associated with metabolic disorders and promote long-term well-being.

1. Insulin's Crucial Role

Insulin, a hormone produced by the pancreas, facilitates the uptake of glucose into cells for energy. Excessive sugar intake over time can lead to a diminished response to insulin, known as insulin resistance.

2. Insulin Resistance Unveiled

Insulin resistance occurs when cells become less responsive to the hormone's signals, leading to elevated blood glucose levels.

The pancreas compensates by producing more insulin, contributing to a cycle of increased insulin levels and resistance.

3. High Sugar Diet as a Precursor

A diet rich in added sugars and refined carbohydrates contributes to the development of insulin resistance. Continuous exposure to high sugar levels prompts cells to downregulate insulin receptors, impairing glucose absorption.

4. Link to Type 2 Diabetes

Prolonged insulin resistance is a primary precursor to type 2 diabetes, a metabolic disorder characterized by chronically elevated blood glucose levels. Individuals with insulin resistance struggle to maintain normal blood sugar levels, increasing the risk of diabetes.

5. Beta-Cell Exhaustion

The pancreas, striving to produce more insulin to overcome resistance, may face exhaustion over time. Beta-cell dysfunction and reduced insulin secretion further contribute to the progression toward diabetes.

6. Role of Inflammation

Chronic inflammation, induced by high sugar consumption, exacerbates insulin resistance. Inflammatory signals interfere with insulin signaling pathways, intensifying the metabolic imbalance.

7. Modifiable Risk Factor

Lifestyle factors, particularly dietary choices, play a pivotal role in the development and progression of insulin resistance. Adopting a low-sugar, balanced diet and incorporating regular physical activity can mitigate this risk.

8. Prevention and Management Strategies

Embracing a whole-food, nutrient-dense diet to promote optimal metabolic health. Engaging in regular physical activity to enhance insulin sensitivity and manage blood sugar levels.

Increased Risk of Cardiovascular Diseases

The modern diet, often laden with excessive sugar, has emerged as a significant contributor to the rising tide of cardiovascular diseases (CVD). Delving into the intricate relationship between sugar consumption and heart health reveals a compelling narrative of increased risks and the importance of mindful dietary choices. Understanding the nexus between excessive sugar consumption and cardiovascular diseases emphasizes the need for proactive lifestyle adjustments. By curbing sugar intake, adopting heart-healthy habits, and prioritizing overall well-being, individuals can actively reduce their risk of developing debilitating cardiovascular conditions.

1. **Elevated Blood Pressure**
High sugar intake is linked to elevated blood pressure, a leading risk factor for cardiovascular diseases. Excessive sugar consumption can contribute to vascular dysfunction and arterial stiffness.

2. **Dyslipidemia and Cholesterol Imbalances**
Sugary diets have been associated with an unfavorable lipid profile, characterized by elevated triglycerides and decreased high-density lipoprotein

(HDL) cholesterol. These lipid imbalances contribute to the development of atherosclerosis, the buildup of plaque in arteries.

3. Insulin Resistance and Metabolic Syndrome

Excessive sugar consumption promotes insulin resistance, a key component of metabolic syndrome. Metabolic syndrome, characterized by insulin resistance, obesity, and other factors, significantly increases the risk of cardiovascular diseases.

4. Inflammation as a Catalyst

Chronic inflammation, triggered by high sugar intake, plays a pivotal role in the development and progression of cardiovascular diseases. Inflammatory processes contribute to the formation of atherosclerotic plaques and increase the vulnerability of blood vessels.

5. Obesity as a Mediator

The association between sugar consumption and obesity is well-established. Obesity, often a consequence of excessive sugar intake, independently elevates the risk of cardiovascular diseases.

6. Endothelial Dysfunction

High sugar levels in the bloodstream can impair endothelial function, affecting the delicate inner lining of blood vessels. Endothelial dysfunction is a precursor to atherosclerosis and other cardiovascular complications.

7. **Platelet Aggregation and Thrombosis**
Sugar-induced inflammation and metabolic disturbances contribute to increased platelet activation and aggregation. These factors enhance the likelihood of blood clot formation, a critical factor in heart attacks and strokes.

8. **Cardiometabolic Health and Lifestyle Choices**
Making informed dietary choices by reducing added sugars and emphasizing heart-healthy foods. Engaging in regular physical activity to promote cardiovascular fitness and mitigate metabolic risk factors.

Promoting Dental Issues

The impact of excessive sugar consumption extends beyond systemic health, casting a shadow on oral well-being. Understanding the detrimental effects of excessive sugar intake on oral health underscores the importance of preventive measures and a sugar-conscious lifestyle. By adopting habits that prioritize oral hygiene and limit sugar exposure, individuals can safeguard their teeth and gums, promoting a lifetime of healthy smiles. Getting to know how sugar promotes dental issues unveils the importance of mindful dietary choices for maintaining a healthy smile.

1. **Formation of Dental Plaque**

Sugars serve as a substrate for the bacteria in the mouth, leading to the formation of dental plaque. Plaque buildup on teeth can result in cavities, gingivitis, and more severe oral health issues.

2. **Acid Production and Tooth Decay**

Oral bacteria ferment sugars, producing acids that demineralize tooth enamel. Repeated exposure to acidic conditions weakens enamel, paving the way for tooth decay and cavities.

3. **Role in Gum Disease**

Sugary diets contribute to the development of gum disease, starting with gingivitis. Persistent inflammation from bacterial action can progress to periodontitis, leading to gum recession and tooth loss.

4. **Promotion of Tooth Erosion**

The acidity resulting from sugar metabolism can contribute to enamel erosion. Weakened enamel makes teeth more susceptible to damage, sensitivity, and discoloration.

5. **Saliva pH Imbalance**

Frequent sugar consumption can disrupt the natural pH balance of saliva. An imbalanced pH creates an environment conducive to bacterial growth and oral health issues.

6. Cariogenic Properties of Added Sugars

Certain sugars, especially sucrose, have been identified as cariogenic, meaning they actively contribute to tooth decay. The adherence of bacteria to teeth increases with the consumption of cariogenic sugars.

7. Dental Health in Children

Early exposure to sugary foods and drinks can lead to a higher risk of developing cavities in children. Establishing healthy dietary habits from a young age is crucial for long-term oral health.

8. Preventive Measures and Oral Hygiene

Practicing regular and effective oral hygiene, including brushing, flossing, and routine dental check-ups. Limiting the intake of added sugars, especially in the form of sugary snacks and beverages. Choosing water over sugary drinks to help maintain oral health.

This comprehensive exploration lays the foundation for individuals to comprehend the multifaceted impact of sugar on their health, motivating them to embark on a transformative journey towards a sugar-free lifestyle.

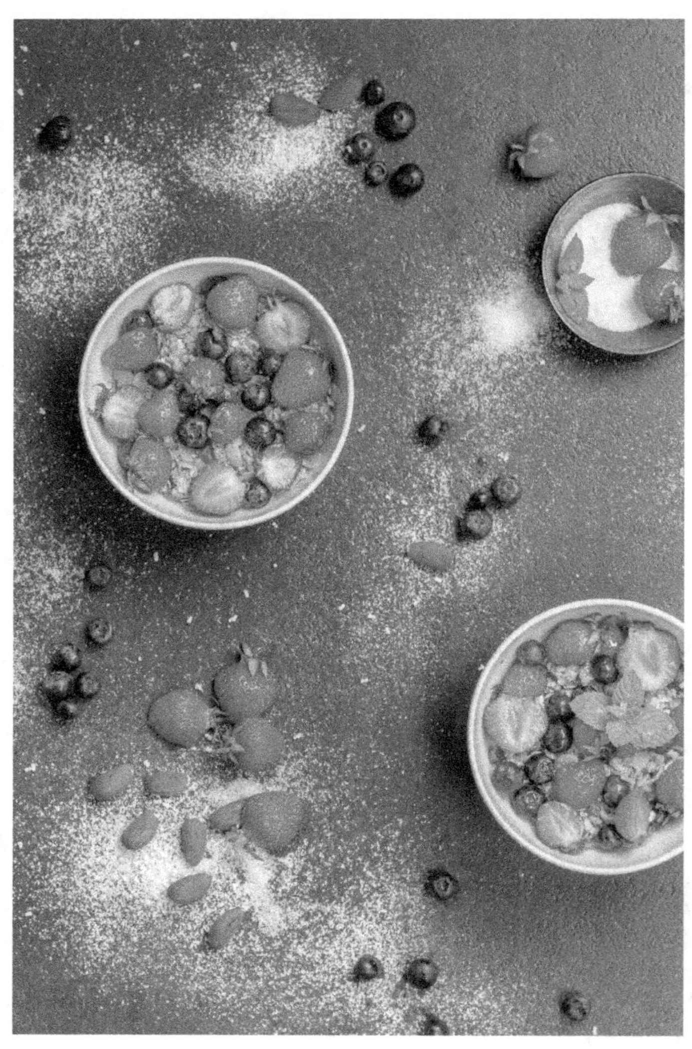

CHAPTER TWO

The Basics of a Sugar-Free Lifestyle.

Navigating a Healthier Dietary Path

Embarking on a sugar-free lifestyle involves more than just eliminating the sweet taste from one's palate. It encompasses a comprehensive approach to nutrition, mindfulness, and conscious food choices. Delving into the basics provides a roadmap for those seeking to transform their health and well-being.

Added Sugar vs. Natural Sugars

Understanding the distinction between added sugars and natural sugars is a cornerstone of making informed dietary choices. This knowledge empowers individuals to navigate the often complex landscape of sweeteners, fostering a healthier relationship with sweetness and overall well-being.

1. Added Sugars

Added sugars are sugars or sweeteners that are incorporated into food and beverages during processing or preparation. They are not naturally present in the original form of the food. Examples include high fructose corn syrup, sucrose (table sugar), honey added to baked goods, and sweetened beverages.

Implications: Consuming excess added sugars is associated with various health risks, including weight gain, insulin resistance, and an increased risk of chronic diseases.

2. Natural Sugars

Natural sugars occur naturally in foods, such as fruits, vegetables, and dairy products. They are inherently present and come packaged with essential nutrients like fiber, vitamins, and minerals. Examples are fructose in fruits, lactose in milk and dairy products, and the natural sugars found in vegetables.

Implications: Natural sugars, when consumed in whole foods, are part of a balanced diet and offer nutritional benefits. The fiber content in many natural sugar sources helps regulate blood sugar levels and supports overall digestive health.

Understanding Added Sugar Labels

Recognizing added sugars on food labels can be challenging due to various names used to disguise them (e.g., sucrose, high fructose corn syrup, agave nectar). Nutrition labels provide valuable information to identify the presence of added sugars in packaged foods.

Health Implications of Excessive Added Sugar Intake

Weight Gain: Added sugars contribute to excess calorie intake, leading to weight gain and obesity.

Metabolic Impact: Excessive added sugar consumption is linked to insulin resistance, metabolic syndrome, and an increased risk of type 2 diabetes.

Cardiovascular Health: High added sugar intake is associated with elevated blood pressure, dyslipidemia, and an increased risk of cardiovascular diseases.

Dental Issues: Added sugars contribute to tooth decay and gum disease by providing fuel for harmful oral bacteria.

Balancing Natural Sugars in a Whole-Food Diet

Whole Foods: Consuming natural sugars in the form of whole foods provides a balance of nutrients, fiber, and antioxidants that contribute to overall health.

Moderation: While natural sugars are part of a balanced diet, moderation is essential to prevent overconsumption.

Making Informed Choices

Reading Labels: Developing the habit of reading food labels to identify and limit added sugars.

Choosing Whole Foods: Prioritizing whole, unprocessed foods rich in natural sugars for a nutrient-dense diet.

Educating Yourself: Staying informed about the different names and sources of added sugars empowers individuals to make healthier choices.

Distinguishing between added sugars and natural sugars involves a nuanced understanding of food composition and label interpretation. By prioritizing whole, nutrient-dense foods and minimizing reliance on processed options, individuals can strike a balance that supports both sweet cravings and overall health.

Overcoming Sugar Cravings

Strategies for a Sweet Victory

Taming the sweet tooth and overcoming sugar cravings is a common challenge on the journey to a healthier lifestyle. Implementing effective strategies can help individuals break free from the cycle of craving and consuming excessive sugars, promoting a balanced and mindful approach to nutrition.

1. Gradual Reduction and Moderation

Baby Steps: Instead of going cold turkey, gradually reduce sugar intake to allow taste buds and cravings to adjust over time.

Moderation: Allowing occasional indulgences in moderation can prevent feelings of deprivation and help in sustaining a long-term sugar-conscious lifestyle.

2. Balancing Macronutrients

Protein and Healthy Fats: Including adequate protein and healthy fats in meals promotes satiety, reducing the likelihood of sudden sugar cravings.

Balanced Meals: Combining carbohydrates with proteins and fats creates a more balanced meal that supports stable blood sugar levels.

3. Hydrating with Water

Thirst vs. Hunger: Staying well-hydrated helps differentiate between true hunger and dehydration, reducing the tendency to reach for sugary snacks.

Infused Water: Infusing water with fruits or herbs can provide a subtle, natural sweetness without added sugars.

4. Choosing Whole Foods

Fruits and Vegetables: Opting for whole fruits and vegetables can satisfy sweet cravings while providing essential nutrients, fiber, and antioxidants.

Complex Carbohydrates: Choosing whole grains and complex carbohydrates provides a more sustained release of energy, reducing the desire for quick sugary fixes.

5. **Mindful Eating Practices**

Savoring Flavors: Taking time to savor each bite and appreciate flavors can enhance the satisfaction derived from meals, reducing the craving for additional sweetness.

Avoiding Distractions: Eating without distractions and being present during meals fosters mindfulness, helping individuals tune in to hunger and fullness cues.

6. **Meal Planning and Preparation**

Preventing Impulse Choices: Planning meals and snacks in advance reduces the likelihood of succumbing to impulsive, sugary choices.

Healthy Snack Options: Having readily available, healthy snack options curbs the temptation to reach for sugary convenience foods.

7. **Cognitive Behavioral Techniques**

Identifying Triggers: Understanding the emotional and situational triggers for sugar cravings allows individuals to develop healthier coping mechanisms.

Positive Reinforcement: Rewarding oneself for making mindful food choices reinforces positive behaviors and helps break the cycle of relying on sugary rewards.

8. **Regular Physical Activity**

Stress Reduction: Engaging in regular physical activity helps manage stress, a common trigger for sugar cravings.

Mood Enhancement: Exercise releases endorphins, which can positively impact mood and reduce the desire for sugary comfort foods.

9. **Sleep Prioritization**

Impact on Cravings: Prioritizing sufficient and quality sleep supports overall well-being and helps regulate hormones that influence hunger and cravings.

Establishing a Routine: Creating a consistent sleep routine enhances the body's natural ability to regulate appetite and cravings.

10. **Seeking Support and Accountability**

Community or Buddy System: Joining a supportive community or partnering with a friend can provide encouragement and accountability on the journey to overcoming sugar cravings.

Professional Guidance: Seeking guidance from a nutritionist or healthcare professional can offer personalized strategies for managing cravings and adopting a balanced diet.

Overcoming sugar cravings is a gradual process that involves a combination of behavioral changes, mindful eating, and a holistic approach to well-being. By incorporating these strategies, individuals can foster a healthier relationship with sweets and pave the way for sustained success in adopting a sugar-conscious lifestyle.

By embracing these basics, individuals can transition to a sugar-free lifestyle with intention and practicality. It's not just about what is excluded from the diet but about the wealth of health-promoting choices that are included, ultimately leading to enhanced well-being and vitality.

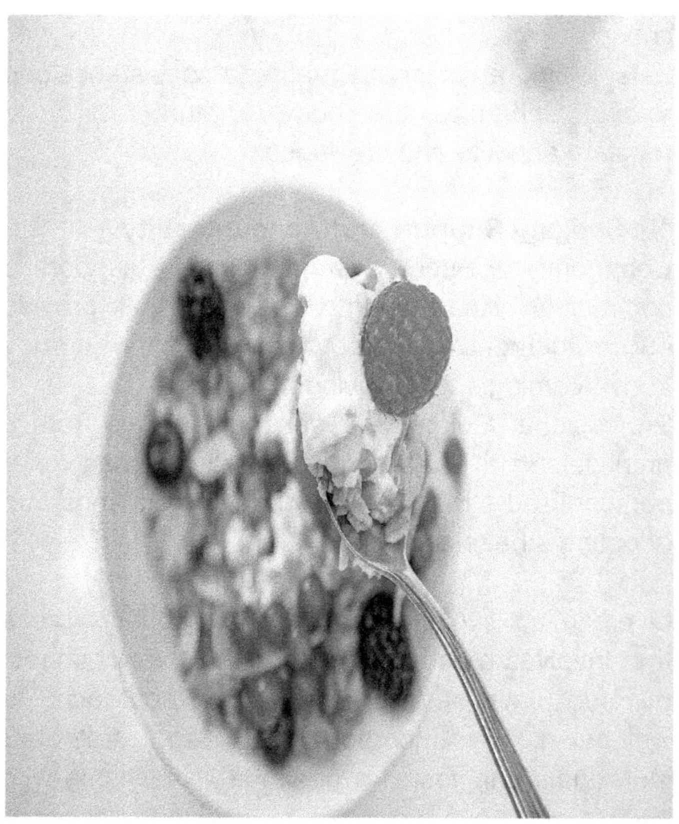

CHAPTER THREE

Sugar-Free Recipes for Every Meal

These sugar-free recipes showcase the diversity and deliciousness that can be achieved without added sugars. By focusing on whole, unprocessed ingredients and embracing natural flavors, individuals can savor a wide range of meals while maintaining a sugar-conscious lifestyle.

Crafting Culinary Delights without the Sweet Stuff

Adopting a sugar-free lifestyle doesn't mean sacrificing flavor or culinary creativity. With mindful ingredient choices and innovative substitutions, it's possible to create delicious, satisfying meals that align with a sugar-conscious approach. Here's a comprehensive guide to sugar-free recipes spanning breakfast, lunch, dinner, and even delightful snacks.

Breakfast

Breakfast Delights: Energizing Morning Options to Kickstart Your Day

Fueling your morning with a nutritious and energizing breakfast is a key ingredient for a successful day. Whether you prefer a quick grab-and-go option or a leisurely sit-down meal, these breakfast delights offer a variety of choices to suit every taste and lifestyle.

1. Classic Overnight Oats
Ingredients: Rolled oats, milk (dairy or plant-based), chia seeds, fruits.
Method: Mix ingredients in a jar, refrigerate overnight, and wake up to a ready-to-eat, fiber-packed delight.

2. Avocado Toast with Poached Egg
Ingredients: Whole-grain toast, ripe avocado, poached egg, salt, pepper.
Method: Spread avocado on toast, top with a poached egg, and season to taste for a protein-rich and satisfying breakfast.

3. Greek Yogurt Parfait
Ingredients: Greek yogurt, granola, mixed berries, honey (optional).

Method: Layer yogurt, granola, and berries in a glass for a delightful and protein-packed parfait.

4. Smoked Salmon Bagel

Ingredients: Whole-grain bagel, smoked salmon, cream cheese, capers, red onion.
Method: Assemble ingredients for a savory and protein-rich breakfast.

5. Homemade Smoothie Bowl

Ingredients: Frozen fruits, spinach, yogurt, toppings (nuts, seeds, granola).
Method: Blend ingredients and top with favorite crunchy toppings for a refreshing and nutrient-packed bowl.

6. Vegetable Omelette

Ingredients: Eggs, bell peppers, onions, tomatoes, spinach, cheese (optional).
Method: Whisk eggs, sauté veggies, add cheese if desired, and fold into an omelette for a customizable and protein-rich breakfast.

7. Whole Grain Pancakes with Berries

Ingredients: Whole-grain pancake mix, water or milk, mixed berries.

Method: Prepare pancakes, top with fresh berries, and drizzle with a touch of honey for a wholesome and satisfying breakfast.

8. Peanut Butter Banana Toast
Ingredients: Whole-grain bread, peanut butter, banana slices.
Method: Spread peanut butter on toast, top with banana slices, and enjoy a combination of protein and natural sweetness.

9. Fruit and Nut Yogurt Bowl
Ingredients: Yogurt, mixed fruits (berries, kiwi, mango), nuts (almonds, walnuts).
Method: Combine yogurt with fresh fruits and nuts for a balanced and crunchy delight.

10. Veggie Breakfast Burrito
Ingredients: Whole-grain tortilla, scrambled eggs, black beans, salsa, avocado.
Method: Assemble ingredients into a burrito for a savory and protein-packed breakfast.

11. Cottage Cheese and Pineapple Bowl
Ingredients: Cottage cheese, fresh pineapple chunks.
Method: Pair protein-rich cottage cheese with juicy pineapple for a quick and refreshing breakfast.

12. **Homemade Acai Bowl**

Ingredients: Frozen acai puree, banana, berries, granola, coconut flakes.

Method: Blend acai with banana and top with granola and berries for a tropical and antioxidant-rich breakfast.

13. **Chia Seed Pudding**

Ingredients: Vanilla extract, chia seeds, and unsweetened almond milk.

Method: Mix ingredients and refrigerate overnight. Top with fresh berries or unsweetened coconut flakes.

Choose a breakfast delight that aligns with your taste preferences and dietary needs, and kickstart your day with the energy and nutrients needed for optimal performance and well-being.

Lunch

Lunchtime Bliss: Nourishing Midday Meals for Sustained Energy and Satisfaction

Lunch is an opportune moment to refuel your body, providing the nutrients needed to power through the remainder of the day. These nourishing and delightful lunch options offer a mix of flavors, textures, and nutrients, ensuring a satisfying midday break.

1. Quinoa Salad with Chickpeas
Ingredients: Cooked quinoa, chickpeas, cherry tomatoes, cucumber, feta cheese, olive oil, lemon juice.
Method: Toss ingredients together for a protein-packed and refreshing quinoa salad.

2. Grilled Chicken Wrap
Ingredients: Grilled chicken, whole-grain wrap, mixed greens, hummus, tomatoes.
Method: Assemble ingredients into a wrap for a balanced and portable lunch.

3. Vegetarian Buddha Bowl
Ingredients: Brown rice or quinoa, roasted vegetables (sweet potatoes, broccoli, carrots), avocado, tahini dressing.
Method: Arrange components in a bowl for a colorful and nutrient-rich lunch.

4. Mediterranean Chickpea Salad
Ingredients: Chickpeas, cherry tomatoes, cucumber, red onion, olives, feta cheese, olive oil.

Method: Combine ingredients for a Mediterranean-inspired salad that's both flavorful and filling.

5. Salmon and Avocado Sushi Bowl

Ingredients: Sushi rice, cooked salmon, avocado slices, seaweed, soy sauce.

Method: Arrange ingredients in a bowl for a deconstructed sushi experience.

6. Quinoa-Stuffed Bell Peppers

Ingredients: Quinoa, black beans, corn, tomatoes, taco seasoning, bell peppers.

Method: Stuff bell peppers with a quinoa and veggie mixture for a satisfying and nutritious lunch.

7. Caprese Sandwich

Ingredients: Whole-grain bread, fresh mozzarella, tomatoes, basil leaves, balsamic glaze.

Method: Assemble ingredients for a classic and refreshing Caprese sandwich.

8. Sweet Potato and Black Bean Burrito Bowl

Ingredients: Roasted sweet potatoes, black beans, brown rice, salsa, guacamole.

Method: Combine ingredients for a hearty and flavorful burrito bowl.

9. Spinach and Feta Stuffed Chicken Breast

Ingredients: Chicken breast, spinach, feta cheese, garlic, lemon.

Method: Stuff chicken breast with a mixture of spinach and feta, then bake for a protein-packed lunch.

10. Vegetable Stir-Fry with Tofu

Ingredients: Tofu, broccoli, bell peppers, snap peas, soy sauce, ginger.

Method: Sauté tofu and veggies, add soy sauce and ginger for a quick and nutritious stir-fry.

11. Chickpea and Kale Caesar Salad

Ingredients: Chickpeas, kale, cherry tomatoes, Parmesan cheese, Caesar dressing.

Method: Toss ingredients for a satisfying and nutrient-dense Caesar salad.

12. Eggplant and Hummus Wrap

Ingredients: Grilled eggplant, whole-grain wrap, hummus, tomatoes, cucumbers.

Method: Assemble ingredients into a wrap for a plant-powered and flavorful lunch.

These lunchtime delights provide a balance of essential nutrients to keep you energized and focused throughout the afternoon. Mix and match based on your preferences, and savor the satisfaction that comes with nourishing your body with wholesome and delicious midday meals.

Dinner

Dinner Creations: Wholesome and Satisfying Dishes for Culinary Delight

As the day winds down, dinner becomes a moment to unwind, nourish the body, and enjoy a flavorful meal. These wholesome and satisfying dinner options offer a variety of tastes, textures, and nutrients, turning your evening meal into a delightful culinary experience.

1. **Baked Lemon Herb Chicken**
  Ingredients: Chicken breasts, lemon, garlic, rosemary, thyme.
Method: Marinate chicken with herbs and bake for a succulent and aromatic main course.

2. **Vegetarian Lentil and Vegetable Stew**
Ingredients: Lentils, carrots, celery, tomatoes, vegetable broth, herbs.

Method: Simmer ingredients for a hearty and nutritious vegetarian stew.

3. Grilled Shrimp and Quinoa Bowl

Ingredients: Grilled shrimp, quinoa, roasted vegetables, avocado, cilantro.

Method: Assemble components in a bowl for a protein-packed and satisfying dinner.

4. Pesto Zoodles with Cherry Tomatoes

Ingredients: Zucchini noodles, cherry tomatoes, homemade basil pesto.

Method: Toss zoodles with pesto and tomatoes for a low-carb and vibrant pasta alternative.

5. Stuffed Bell Peppers with Turkey and Quinoa

Ingredients: Black beans, salsa, quinoa, ground turkey, and bell peppers

Method: Fill peppers with a mixture of turkey, quinoa, and black beans, then bake for a wholesome and colorful dish.

6. Salmon and Asparagus Foil Packets

Ingredients: Salmon fillets, asparagus, lemon, dill.

Method: Create individual foil packets with salmon and asparagus, then bake for a quick and flavorful dinner.

7. Mushroom and Spinach Risotto

Ingredients: Arborio rice, mushrooms, spinach, vegetable broth, Parmesan cheese.

Method: Cook a creamy risotto with sautéed mushrooms and wilted spinach for a comforting meal.

8. Cauliflower and Chickpea Curry

Ingredients: Cauliflower, chickpeas, coconut milk, curry spices.

Method: Simmer ingredients in a flavorful curry sauce for a vegetarian-friendly and satisfying dinner.

9. Spaghetti Squash Bolognese

Ingredients: Spaghetti squash, lean ground beef or turkey, tomato sauce, herbs.

Method: Roast spaghetti squash and top with a hearty Bolognese sauce for a low-carb twist on a classic.

10. Stir-Fried Tofu and Broccoli

Ingredients: Tofu, broccoli, bell peppers, soy sauce, ginger.

Method: Sauté tofu and veggies with soy sauce and ginger for a quick and nutritious stir-fry.

11. Chicken and Vegetable Skewers with Chimichurri Sauce

Ingredients: Chicken breast, bell peppers, onions, cherry tomatoes, chimichurri sauce.

Method: Thread ingredients onto skewers, grill, and serve with zesty chimichurri sauce for a flavorful dinner.

12. Sweet Potato and Black Bean Enchiladas

Ingredients: Sweet potatoes, black beans, whole-grain tortillas, enchilada sauce.

Method: Roll sweet potatoes and black beans in tortillas, top with enchilada sauce, and bake for a satisfying and plant-powered dinner.

13. Baked Salmon with Lemon Herb Sauce

Ingredients: Salmon fillets, lemon, garlic, herbs.

Method: Bake salmon with a lemon herb sauce for a flavorful and low-carb dinner.

14. Zucchini Noodles with Pesto

Ingredients: Zucchini noodles, homemade basil pesto.

Method: Spiralize zucchini, toss with pesto, and top with pine nuts for a light and satisfying pasta alternative.

15. **Cauliflower Crust Pizza**
Ingredients: Cauliflower, mozzarella, eggs, pizza toppings.
Method: Blend cauliflower, mix with cheese and eggs, bake, and add favorite pizza toppings for a guilt-free pizza night.

These dinner creations bring a mix of vibrant colors, flavors, and nutritional benefits to your evening table. Experiment with these recipes to find the perfect balance of taste and nourishment that suits your culinary preferences.

Snacks

Snack Attack: Guilt-Free Treats for Satisfying Cravings

When the urge for a snack strikes, it's possible to indulge in delicious treats without compromising your commitment to a healthy lifestyle. These guilt-free snack options provide a perfect balance of flavor, nutrition, and satisfaction to curb cravings without the guilt.

1. Greek Yogurt and Berry Parfait

Ingredients: Greek yogurt, a mixture of berries, and a honey drizzle are the ingredients.

Method: Layer yogurt with fresh berries and honey for a protein-packed and naturally sweet parfait.

2. Roasted Chickpeas

Ingredients: Canned chickpeas, olive oil, spices (paprika, cumin, garlic powder).

Method: Toss chickpeas in spices and roast for a crunchy and protein-rich snack.

3. Nut Butter and Banana Rice Cakes

Ingredients: Brown rice cakes, nut butter (almond, peanut), banana slices.

Method: Spread nut butter on rice cakes, top with banana slices for a satisfying and wholesome treat.

4. Dark Chocolate-Covered Almonds

Ingredients: Dark chocolate, raw almonds.

Method: Melt dark chocolate, coat almonds, and let them cool for a decadent and antioxidant-rich snack.

5. Vegetable Sticks with Hummus

Ingredients: Carrot, cucumber, bell pepper sticks, hummus.

Method: Dip fresh vegetable sticks into hummus for a crunchy and fiber-packed snack.

6. Kale Chips

Ingredients: Fresh kale, olive oil, sea salt.

Method: Toss kale in olive oil, sprinkle with sea salt, and bake until crispy for a nutrient-dense and flavorful chip alternative.

7. Fruit Salad with Mint

Ingredients: Assorted fruits (watermelon, berries, kiwi), fresh mint.

Method: Combine fruits and mint for a refreshing and hydrating snack.

8. Cottage Cheese and Pineapple Salsa

Ingredients: Cottage cheese, fresh pineapple, lime juice.

Method: Top cottage cheese with diced pineapple and a squeeze of lime for a tropical and protein-rich delight.

9. Trail Mix with Nuts and Seeds

Ingredients: Almonds, walnuts, pumpkin seeds, dried cranberries.

Method: Mix nuts and seeds for a satisfying and energy-boosting trail mix.

10. Edamame with Sea Salt

Ingredients: Edamame (steamed or boiled), sea salt.
Method: Sprinkle steamed edamame with sea salt for a protein-packed and easy-to-eat snack.

11. Rice Cake with Avocado

Ingredients: Brown rice cake, mashed avocado, a sprinkle of black pepper.
Method: Spread mashed avocado on a rice cake, add a dash of pepper for a quick and satiating snack.

12. Yogurt-Dipped Frozen Grapes

Ingredients: Grapes, Greek yogurt.
Method: Dip grapes in Greek yogurt, freeze until solid for a refreshing and sweet frozen treat.

13. Apple Slices with Nut Butter

Ingredients: Apple slices, nut butter (almond, peanut)
Method: Spread nut butter on apple slices for a delightful combination of sweetness and protein.

14. **Chia Seed Pudding Cups**

Ingredients: Chia seeds, almond milk, vanilla extract.

Method: Mix ingredients, refrigerate until set, and portion into cups for a nutrient-rich and satisfying pudding.

15. **Avocado and Salsa Dip**

Ingredients: Avocado, tomatoes, onions, lime juice.

Method: Mash avocado, mix with diced veggies, and enjoy with cucumber or celery sticks.

16. **Spiced Almonds**

Ingredients: Almonds, cinnamon, nutmeg.

Method: Toss almonds in spices and bake for a crunchy, sweet-free snack.

17. **Cheese and Veggie Skewers**

Ingredients: Cherry tomatoes, mozzarella, basil.

Method: Thread ingredients onto skewers for a refreshing and satisfying snack.

Indulge in these guilt-free treats whenever the snack attack strikes, knowing that you're nourishing your body with wholesome ingredients and satisfying your taste buds without compromising on health.

Desserts

1. Berry and Coconut Cream Parfait

Ingredients: Mixed berries, coconut cream.
Method: Layer berries with coconut cream for a naturally sweet and creamy dessert.

2. Dark Chocolate Covered Strawberries

Ingredients: Dark chocolate, fresh strawberries.
Method: Melt dark chocolate, dip strawberries, and let them cool for a simple, sweet treat.

3. Baked Apple with Cinnamon

Ingredients: Apple, cinnamon.
Method: Core an apple, sprinkle with cinnamon, and bake for a warm and comforting dessert.

CHAPTER FOUR

Weight Strategies Without Sacrificing Flavor

Embarking on a weight-loss journey doesn't mean bidding farewell to delicious and satisfying meals. By incorporating mindful strategies into your culinary approach, you can enjoy flavorful dishes that not only tantalize your taste buds but also support your wellness goals.

1. Embrace Whole Foods

Prioritize fresh, whole foods like fruits, vegetables, lean proteins, and whole grains. These nutrient-dense options provide essential vitamins and minerals while contributing to satiety.

2. Balanced Plate Method

Aim for a well-balanced plate by incorporating lean proteins, colorful vegetables, whole grains, and healthy fats. This approach not only enhances nutritional intake but also promotes a feeling of fullness.

3. **Mindful Portion Control**

Pay attention to portion proportions to prevent overindulging. Utilize smaller plates, pay attention to your body's signals of hunger, and mindfully enjoy every mouthful.

4. **Flavorful Herbs and Spices**

Enhance the taste of your meals with herbs and spices instead of excessive salt, sugar, or unhealthy fats. Experiment with a variety of seasonings to add depth and complexity to your dishes.

5. **Healthy Cooking Methods**

Use less oil while grilling, baking, steaming, or sautéing as healthier cooking techniques. These methods retain the flavors of ingredients without adding unnecessary calories.

6. **Smart Substitutions**

Make smart ingredient substitutions without sacrificing taste. For example, use Greek yogurt instead of sour cream, whole-grain options instead of refined grains, and lean proteins in place of fatty cuts.

7. **Explore Plant-Based Options**

Integrate plant-based meals into your repertoire. Plant-based diets can be flavorful and satisfying while often being lower in calories and saturated fats.

8. Hydration with Infused Water

Stay hydrated with infused water flavored with herbs, fruits, or cucumbers. This not only adds a burst of flavor but also helps control appetite.

9. Strategic Meal Timing

Plan meals and snacks strategically throughout the day to maintain steady energy levels. Include a balance of macronutrients to keep hunger at bay.

10. Preparation Techniques

Experiment with various cooking techniques like marinating, roasting, or slow cooking to enhance natural flavors without relying on excessive fats or sugars.

11. DIY Dressings and Sauces

Prepare homemade dressings and sauces using fresh ingredients. This allows you to control the ingredients, avoiding hidden sugars and unnecessary additives.

12. **High-Fiber Choices**

- Choose high-fiber foods like beans, legumes, and whole grains. Fiber-rich meals contribute to a feeling of fullness, reducing the likelihood of overeating.

13. **Protein-Packed Snacks**

Opt for protein-packed snacks between meals. Greek yogurt, nuts, and seeds are tasty options that can help control cravings.

14. **Colorful and Diverse Produce**

Explore a variety of colorful fruits and vegetables. Not only do they bring vibrancy to your plate, but they also provide a spectrum of nutrients.

15. **Enjoying Moderation**

Allow yourself occasional indulgences in moderation. Depriving yourself of treats entirely may lead to cravings, so savoring small portions of your favorite foods can be part of a sustainable approach.

By integrating these weight-loss strategies into your culinary routine, you can navigate towards a healthier lifestyle without compromising on the joy of delicious and flavorful meals. It's about savoring the journey to wellness, one tasty and nutritious bite at a time.

Understanding the Link Between Sugar and Weight Gain

The relationship between sugar consumption and weight gain is a complex interplay that extends beyond simple caloric intake. Exploring this connection provides valuable insights into how sugar affects our bodies and influences the scale.

1. Caloric Density

While sugar itself contributes calories to the diet, its high caloric density means that even small amounts can add up quickly. Consuming sugary beverages and snacks without awareness can lead to an excess of calories.

2. Insulin Resistance

High sugar intake can contribute to insulin resistance, where cells become less responsive to insulin's signal. This can result in increased fat storage, particularly around the abdominal area.

3. Leptin Resistance

Leptin is a hormone that regulates hunger and signals feelings of fullness. Excessive sugar consumption may lead to leptin resistance, disrupting the body's ability to recognize when it's satisfied, potentially leading to overeating.

4. **Promotes Fat Storage**

Excess sugar, especially fructose found in high-fructose corn syrup, can stimulate the liver to convert sugar into fat. This contributes to increased fat accumulation, particularly in the liver, which is associated with weight gain.

5. **Highly Palatable Foods**

Foods high in sugar are often highly palatable, triggering reward centers in the brain. This can lead to overconsumption as individuals seek the pleasurable sensations associated with sugary treats.

6. **Empty Calories**

Sugary foods and beverages often provide "empty calories" with little to no nutritional value. Consuming these empty calories may lead to nutrient deficiencies as individuals may replace nutrient-dense foods with sugary options.

7. Sugar and Belly Fat

Excessive sugar intake, particularly in the form of added sugars and sugary beverages, is linked to the accumulation of visceral fat—fat stored around internal organs. This type of fat is associated with various health risks, including metabolic syndrome and cardiovascular issues.

8. Increased Appetite

Eating sugary meals might cause blood sugar levels to jump quickly and then plummet. This cycle may trigger increased hunger and cravings, contributing to overeating and weight gain over time.

9. Disruption of Hormonal Balance

Sugar can influence hormones involved in appetite regulation, such as ghrelin and insulin. These hormone imbalances can interfere with the body's normal processes for controlling weight.

10. Role of Fructose

Fructose, a component of sugar, is metabolized in the liver, potentially leading to the accumulation of fat. High intake of fructose, often found in sugary beverages and processed foods, is associated with adverse metabolic effects.

11. **Impact on Metabolism**

Excessive sugar intake may contribute to metabolic dysfunction, impairing the body's ability to burn calories efficiently and increasing the likelihood of weight gain.

12. **Inflammatory Response**

High sugar consumption can contribute to chronic inflammation, which is linked to various health issues, including obesity. Chronic inflammation can interfere with metabolic processes, potentially promoting weight gain.

Understanding the intricate relationship between sugar and weight gain is crucial for making informed dietary choices. By adopting a balanced and mindful approach to sugar intake, individuals can contribute to their overall well-being and maintain a healthy weight.

Portion Control Tips for Effective Weight Management

Maintaining a healthy weight involves not just what you eat but also how much you eat. Portion control is a key aspect of a balanced diet, promoting mindful consumption and preventing overindulgence. Here are practical tips to help you master portion control for effective weight management:

1. Use Smaller Plates

Opt for smaller plates to create the illusion of a fuller plate, making it easier to feel satisfied with smaller portions.

2. Divide Your Plate

Visualize your plate divided into sections: fill half with vegetables, a quarter with lean protein, and the remaining quarter with whole grains or starchy vegetables. This promotes a balanced and portion-controlled meal.

3. Mindful Eating

Slow down and savor each bite. Paying attention to your meal can help you recognize when you're full, preventing overeating.

4. Pre-Portion Snacks

Divide snacks into single-serving portions to avoid mindlessly eating from larger containers. This is especially effective for nuts, fruits, and other snack items.

5. Measure Ingredients

Use measuring cups, spoons, or a kitchen scale to portion out ingredients accurately, especially when cooking or baking.

6. Beware of Liquid Calories

Be mindful of portion sizes with beverages, including sugary drinks and alcohol. Consider using smaller glasses or diluting drinks to reduce calorie intake.

7. Listen to Hunger Cues

Eat when you're hungry and stop when you're satisfied. Tune into your body's signals rather than finishing what's on your plate.

8. Be Wary of Restaurant Portions

Restaurant servings are often larger than necessary. Consider sharing a dish, asking for a to-go box at the beginning of the meal, or choosing smaller portions if available.

9. Single-Serve Packages

Opt for single-serving packages when buying snacks or treats. This helps control portion sizes and prevents overindulgence.

10. Plate Leftovers Before Eating

- When serving meals, plate your food rather than bringing serving dishes to the table. This makes it less tempting to go for seconds.

11. Choose Nutrient-Dense Foods

Prioritize nutrient-dense foods that offer more vitamins, minerals, and fiber per calorie. This allows you to eat satisfying portions while meeting nutritional needs.

12. **Practice the Half-Plate Rule**

When dining out, follow the "half-plate rule" by requesting half of your meal to be boxed up before it's served, ensuring you eat a reasonable portion.

13. **Visualize Portion Sizes**

Familiarize yourself with portion sizes using visual cues. For example, a serving of meat is about the size of a deck of cards, and a cup of vegetables is roughly the size of a baseball.

14. **Stay Hydrated**

Drink water before meals to help you feel fuller and avoid overeating. Sometimes, thirst is confused with hunger.

15. **Plan Balanced Snacks**

When snacking, combine protein, fiber, and healthy fats for a satisfying and portion-controlled option. Examples include apple slices with peanut butter or Greek yogurt with berries.

Mastering portion control is a powerful tool in achieving and maintaining a healthy weight. By incorporating these tips into your daily routine, you can strike a balance between enjoying your favorite foods and ensuring that your portions align with your wellness goals.

Incorporating Exercise for Lasting Results: Building a Sustainable Fitness Routine

Achieving and maintaining a healthy weight goes hand in hand with regular physical activity. Exercise not only aids in weight management but also contributes to overall well-being. Here's a guide to incorporating exercise into your lifestyle for lasting results:

1. **Set Realistic Goals:** Define achievable and realistic fitness goals. Whether it's walking 10,000 steps a day, jogging for 20 minutes, or attending a weekly fitness class, setting attainable milestones keeps you motivated.

2. **Find Activities You Enjoy**: Experiment with different types of exercise until you find activities you genuinely enjoy. Whether it's dancing, cycling, swimming, or hiking, making fitness enjoyable increases the likelihood of maintaining a routine.

3. **Make It a Routine**: Establish a consistent workout routine. Treat exercise like any other appointment, scheduling it into your calendar. This helps create a habit and makes it less likely to be overlooked.

4. **Mix Cardio and Strength Training**: Combine cardiovascular exercises, like running or cycling, with strength training. Strength training builds lean

muscle mass, which can boost metabolism and contribute to long-term weight management.

5. **Start Gradually**: If you're new to exercise or returning after a hiatus, start slowly to avoid burnout or injury. As you get more fit, gradually up the intensity and length of your workouts.

6. **Incorporate Daily Acti**vity: Integrate physical activity into your daily life. Take the stairs, walk or bike to nearby destinations, or engage in household chores that involve movement. These small activities add up over time.

7. **Explore Group Fitness**: Joining group fitness classes or sports teams can make exercise more enjoyable and provide a sense of community. The social aspect can motivate you to stick with your routine.

8. **Set Realistic Time Commitment**s: Recognize that not every workout needs to be lengthy. Short, high-intensity sessions or even a brisk walk during your lunch break can contribute to overall fitness.

9. **Prioritize Consistency Over Intensity**: Consistency is key. Aim for regular, moderate-intensity exercise rather than sporadic, intense workouts. Building a sustainable routine is more important than occasional bursts of activity.

10. **Include Flexibility and Balance Exercises:** Incorporate flexibility and balance exercises into your routine. Activities like yoga or Pilates not only enhance flexibility but also contribute to overall body strength.

11. **Set Weekly Activity Goals:** Establish weekly activity goals to ensure you stay on track. Whether it's a certain number of workouts, total minutes of exercise, or specific fitness achievements, these goals provide a sense of direction.

12. **Invest in Wearable Fitness Tech**: Consider using wearable fitness technology to track your activity levels. Devices like fitness trackers or smartwatches can provide insights into your daily movement and motivate you to meet your goals.

13. **Get Professional Guidance**: Consult with a fitness professional or personal trainer to create a personalized exercise plan. They can tailor workouts to your fitness level, goals, and any specific considerations.

14. **Vary Your Routine**: Keep things interesting by varying your exercise routine. Trying new activities not only prevents boredom but also challenges different muscle groups, promoting overall fitness.

15. **Celebrate Achievements:** Celebrate milestones and achievements along your fitness journey. Whether it's reaching a certain number of

workouts or mastering a new exercise, acknowledging progress reinforces positive habits.

Incorporating exercise into your lifestyle is a powerful strategy for achieving lasting results in weight management and overall health. By embracing activities you enjoy and gradually building a routine that fits your life, you can cultivate a sustainable approach to fitness that contributes to long-term well-being.

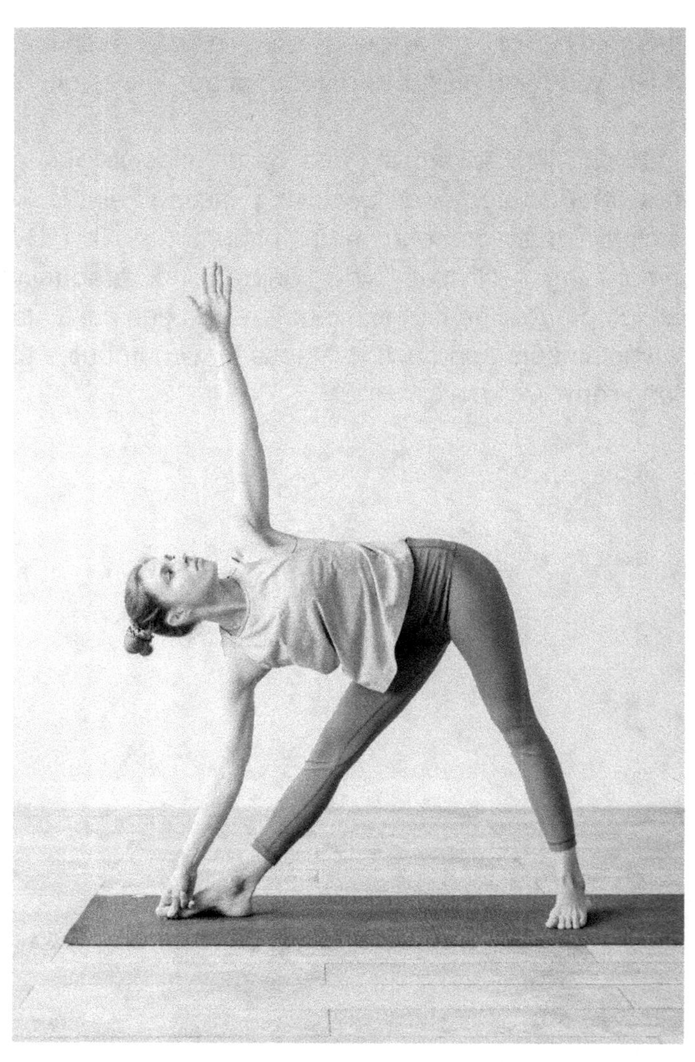

CHAPTER FIVE

Diabetes Management Through Dietary Choices

Effective diabetes management revolves significantly around making informed and mindful dietary choices. Crafting a balanced and tailored eating plan can help stabilize blood sugar levels, improve insulin sensitivity, and enhance overall well-being.

Managing diabetes through dietary choices is a multifaceted journey that requires commitment and a holistic approach. By embracing a nutrient-rich, well-balanced diet, individuals can take significant strides toward better blood sugar control and overall health. Always consult with healthcare professionals for personalized guidance based on your specific needs and medical history.

The Role of Sugar in Diabetes: Unraveling the Glucose Connection

Diabetes is a metabolic disorder characterized by impaired insulin function, leading to elevated blood sugar levels. While the relationship between sugar and diabetes is complex, understanding the role of sugar in this condition is crucial for effective management. Here's a closer look at how sugar influences diabetes:

1. **Types of Diabetes:** There are different types of diabetes, with the most common being Type 1 and Type 2. In Type 1 diabetes, the body doesn't produce insulin, while in Type 2 diabetes, the body either doesn't produce enough insulin or doesn't use it effectively.

2. **Glucose and Insulin Dynamics**: The primary role of insulin, a hormone produced by the pancreas, is to regulate blood sugar (glucose) levels. After consuming carbohydrates, the body breaks them down into glucose, causing a rise in blood sugar. Insulin facilitates the uptake of glucose by cells for energy or storage.

3. **Hyperglycemia in Diabetes:** In diabetes, the regulation of blood sugar is disrupted. In Type 1 diabetes, the absence of insulin prevents glucose absorption by cells, leading to elevated blood sugar levels. In Type 2 diabetes, cells may become insulin resistant, causing a similar outcome.

4. **Impact of Sugars on Blood Sugar Levels:** Sugars, including both natural sugars found in fruits and added sugars in processed foods, can affect blood sugar levels. Simple carbohydrates, like those found in sugary snacks and beverages, can cause rapid spikes in blood glucose.

5. **Glycemic Index and Load**: The glycemic index (GI) and glycemic load (GL) are measures of how quickly a food raises blood sugar. Foods with a high

GI or GL can lead to more significant fluctuations in blood glucose levels. Monitoring and choosing low-GI foods can be beneficial for people with diabetes.

6. **Added Sugars and Insulin Resistance**: Diets high in added sugars have been associated with insulin resistance, a key factor in Type 2 diabetes. Excessive sugar consumption may contribute to the body's reduced responsiveness to insulin, making it challenging to regulate blood sugar effectively.

7. **Fructose and Metabolic Effects**: Fructose, a component of sugar, is metabolized differently than glucose. High intake of fructose, often found in high-fructose corn syrup, has been linked to adverse metabolic effects, including insulin resistance and increased fat accumulation in the liver.

8. **Connection Between Obesity and Type 2 Diabetes:** Excessive sugar intake, particularly in the form of sugary beverages and processed foods, can contribute to weight gain and obesity. Obesity is a significant risk factor for Type 2 diabetes.

9. **Importance of Sugar Monitoring:** People with diabetes often need to monitor their carbohydrate intake, including sugars, to manage blood sugar levels effectively. Regular monitoring helps individuals make informed dietary choices and adjust insulin or medications as needed.

10. **Balancing Sugar Intake**: Balancing sugar intake within the context of a well-rounded, nutrient-dense diet is essential for individuals with diabetes. Emphasizing whole foods, controlling portions, and choosing low-GI options can help stabilize blood sugar levels.

11. **Role of Dietary Fiber:** Dietary fiber, found in fruits, vegetables, and whole grains, can slow down the absorption of sugars and improve blood sugar control. Including fiber-rich foods is an integral part of managing diabetes through diet.

12. **Individual Variability:** The impact of sugar on blood sugar levels can vary among individuals. Factors such as overall diet, physical activity, and individual metabolic responses play a role in determining how different people respond to sugar.

13. **Holistic Diabetes Management**: Effective diabetes management involves a holistic approach, including medication (if prescribed), regular physical activity, and a well-balanced diet. Monitoring and adapting to individual needs are crucial components of this multifaceted strategy.

Understanding the role of sugar in diabetes underscores the importance of making informed dietary choices tailored to individual needs. By fostering a balanced approach to nutrition, individuals with diabetes can work towards better blood sugar control and overall health. Always consult with healthcare professionals for personalized guidance based on specific health conditions and goals.

Creating Balanced Meals for Blood Sugar Control

Maintaining stable blood sugar levels is paramount for individuals managing conditions like diabetes. Crafting balanced meals involves thoughtful consideration of food choices to minimize blood sugar fluctuations. Here's a guide to creating meals that support blood sugar control:

1. **Incorporate Lean Proteins:** Start with a foundation of lean proteins, such as chicken, turkey, fish, tofu, or legumes. Proteins help stabilize blood sugar levels and provide a sense of fullness.

2. **Choose Whole Grains**: Opt for whole grains like quinoa, brown rice, or whole wheat bread. These choices have a lower glycemic index, leading to a slower rise in blood sugar after meals.

3. **Load Up on Non-Starchy Vegetables**: Fill a significant portion of your plate with non-starchy vegetables like leafy greens, broccoli, peppers, and cauliflower. These vegetables are rich in fiber and nutrients without significantly impacting blood sugar.

4. **Incorporate Healthy Fats:** Include healthy fats, such as avocados, nuts, seeds, and olive oil. Fats contribute to satiety and can help slow down the absorption of sugars, promoting stable blood sugar levels.

5. **Moderate Portion Sizes**: Practice portion control to avoid overeating. Using smaller plates and measuring servings can help regulate calorie intake and prevent spikes in blood sugar.

6. **Prioritize Fiber-Rich Foods**: Choose foods high in dietary fiber, including fruits, vegetables, whole grains, and legumes. Fiber aids in digestion, slows down the release of glucose, and contributes to a feeling of fullness.

7. **Mindful Carbohydrate Choices:** Be strategic about carbohydrates by selecting complex carbs with a lower glycemic index. Include sweet potatoes, legumes, and whole grains while minimizing refined and processed carbohydrates.

8. **Balanced Snacks**: Plan balanced snacks that include a mix of protein, fiber, and healthy fats. Examples include Greek yogurt with berries, a handful of nuts with an apple, or carrot sticks with hummus.

9. **Hydrate with Water:** Stay hydrated with water throughout the day. Water supports overall health

and can help control appetite, preventing overconsumption.

10. **Limit Added Sugars:** Minimize added sugars in your meals. Read labels carefully and choose foods and beverages with little to no added sugars.

11. **Include Colorful Produce:** Aim for a variety of colorful fruits and vegetables to ensure a broad spectrum of nutrients. Different colors often indicate distinct vitamins, minerals, and antioxidants.

12. **Spread Meals Throughout the Day:** Aim for regular meals spaced throughout the day to maintain steady blood sugar levels. Avoid prolonged periods without eating to prevent dips or spikes in glucose.

13. **Mindful Meal Timing:** Consider the timing of your meals. Eating at consistent intervals can help regulate blood sugar and support medication management if applicable.

14. **Whole, Unprocessed Foods:** Choose whole, unprocessed foods whenever possible. Minimize reliance on pre-packaged or processed meals, as they may contain hidden sugars and unhealthy fats.

15. **Experiment with Herbs and Spices:** Enhance flavor without added sugars or salt by experimenting with herbs and spices. Seasoning

your meals creatively can make balanced eating more enjoyable.

Creating balanced meals for blood sugar control involves a holistic approach that considers a variety of nutrient-dense foods. By focusing on lean proteins, whole grains, fiber-rich vegetables, and healthy fats, individuals can design meals that promote stable blood sugar levels and contribute to overall well-being. Always consult with healthcare professionals for personalized guidance based on specific health conditions and goals.

Practical Tips for Daily Diabetes Management

Effectively managing diabetes involves a daily commitment to lifestyle choices that support stable blood sugar levels. Incorporating practical strategies into your routine can significantly impact your overall health and well-being. Here are practical tips for daily diabetes management:

1. Monitor your blood sugar levels regularly, as advised by your healthcare team. This empowers you with valuable information to make informed decisions about your diet, physical activity, and medication.

2. Establish a regular meal schedule with balanced portions. Consistency in meal timing can help

regulate blood sugar levels and support medication management.

3. Opt for low-glycemic foods, such as whole grains, legumes, and non-starchy vegetables. These choices have a gentler impact on blood sugar levels.

4. Practice carbohydrate counting to manage your carb intake effectively. This skill is particularly useful for individuals using insulin or other medications that require dosage adjustments based on carbohydrate consumption.

5. Drink plenty of water throughout the day. Proper hydration supports overall health and can help control appetite, preventing excessive snacking.

6. Incorporate regular physical activity into your routine. A combination of strength training, flexibility training, and cardiovascular exercise should be your goal. Consult your healthcare team for personalized recommendations.

7. Structure your meals with a focus on lean proteins, whole grains, non-starchy vegetables, and healthy fats. This well-rounded strategy aids in blood sugar regulation.

8. Practice portion control to manage calorie intake and prevent overeating. Slow down during meals,

chew thoroughly, and pay attention to hunger and fullness cues.

9. If prescribed medications, understand the instructions thoroughly. Take medications as directed by your healthcare provider, and communicate any concerns or challenges you may face.

10. Plan healthy snacks to prevent extreme hunger between meals. Choose options that include protein and fiber to help stabilize blood sugar levels.

11. Incorporate stress-management techniques into your daily routine, such as meditation, deep breathing exercises, or activities that bring joy. Chronic stress can impact blood sugar levels.

12. Schedule regular check-ups with your healthcare team. These appointments allow for comprehensive assessments of your diabetes management plan and adjustments if needed.

13. Pay attention to foot care. Inspect your feet daily for any cuts, bruises, or signs of infection. Diabetes can affect circulation and nerve function, making foot care crucial.

14. Read food labels carefully to identify hidden sugars and make informed choices. Understanding nutritional information supports mindful eating.

15. Prioritize good sleep hygiene. Aim for consistent sleep patterns and quality sleep, as inadequate sleep can affect blood sugar control.

16. Keep a diabetes emergency kit, including glucose-monitoring supplies and snacks, especially if you're prone to hypoglycemia. Be prepared for unexpected situations.

17. Seek support from diabetes education classes, support groups, or online communities. Connecting with others facing similar challenges can provide valuable insights and encouragement.

18. Prioritize regular dental check-ups. Individuals with diabetes are at an increased risk of gum disease, emphasizing the importance of oral health.

19. Be aware of temperature extremes, as extreme heat or cold can impact insulin effectiveness and blood sugar control.

20. Maintain open communication with your healthcare team. Share any concerns, challenges, or changes in your health to ensure your diabetes management plan remains tailored to your needs.

Consistent and proactive daily diabetes management is key to long-term health and well-being. By integrating these practical tips into your routine, you empower yourself to navigate the complexities of diabetes with resilience and confidence. Always consult with your healthcare professionals for personalized advice and adjustments to your management plan.

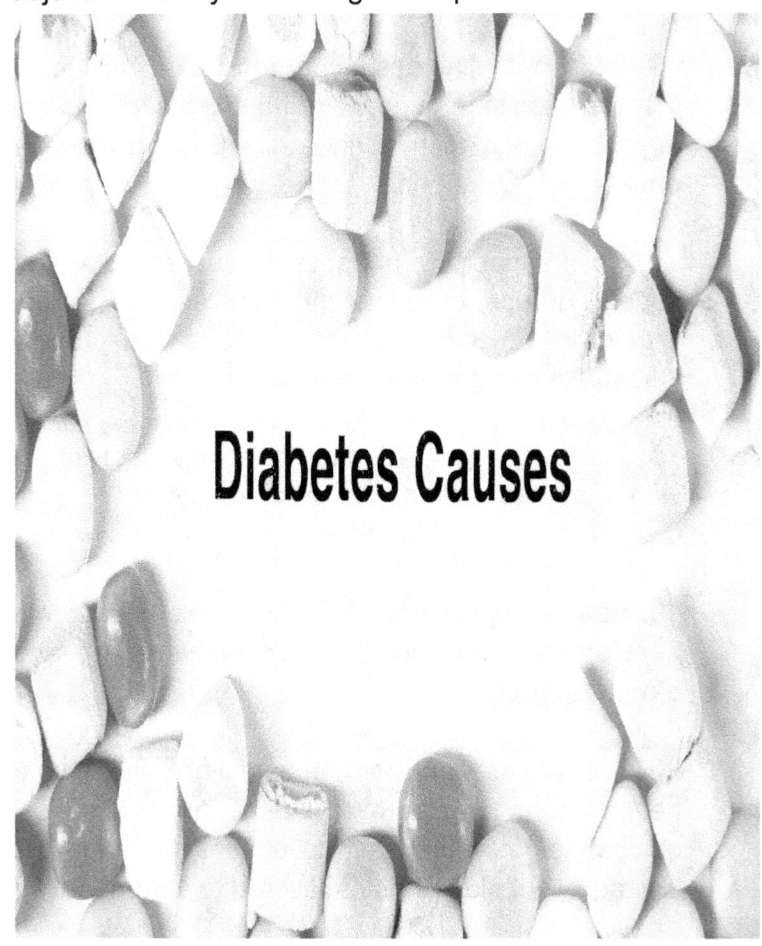

CHAPTER SIX

Lowering Cholesterol Naturally

Maintaining healthy cholesterol levels is essential for cardiovascular well-being. High cholesterol levels, particularly elevated levels of LDL (low-density lipoprotein) cholesterol, can contribute to heart disease. Adopting natural strategies to lower cholesterol is a proactive and sustainable approach to support heart health

The Connection Between Sugar and Cholesterol

Understanding the intricate relationship between sugar and cholesterol is crucial for comprehending the broader impact on cardiovascular health. While dietary sugars themselves do not contain cholesterol, their influence on metabolism and various physiological processes can indirectly affect cholesterol levels. Here's a comprehensive exploration of the connection between sugar and cholesterol:

1. Effect on Triglycerides: Diets high in added sugars, particularly fructose, can contribute to elevated triglyceride levels. Triglycerides are a type of fat in the blood, and high levels are often associated with an increased risk of heart disease.

2. Insulin Resistance and Cholesterol: Excessive sugar intake has been linked to insulin resistance, a condition where cells become less responsive to insulin. Insulin resistance is associated with dyslipidemia—a disruption in lipid (fat) metabolism—resulting in increased levels of LDL (low-density lipoprotein) cholesterol and decreased levels of HDL (high-density lipoprotein) cholesterol.

3. Impact on Lipoproteins: Diets high in refined sugars may influence the composition of lipoproteins, which transport cholesterol in the blood. This can lead to an unfavorable balance, with higher levels of LDL cholesterol, often referred to as "bad" cholesterol.

4. Fructose Metabolism: Fructose, a component of table sugar (sucrose) and high-fructose corn syrup, is metabolized primarily in the liver. Excessive fructose intake has been associated with increased production of triglycerides, leading to higher levels of VLDL (very low-density lipoprotein) cholesterol.

5. Contribution to Weight Gain: Diets rich in sugary foods and beverages are often calorie-dense and can contribute to weight gain and obesity. Excess body weight is a risk factor for dyslipidemia and can negatively impact cholesterol levels.

6. Impact on LDL Particle Size: Some studies suggest that high sugar intake may lead to a shift in

LDL particle size towards smaller, denser particles. Smaller LDL particles are considered more atherogenic, meaning they may contribute to the development of atherosclerosis more readily than larger particles.

7. Inflammatory Response: Excessive sugar consumption may contribute to chronic inflammation, which is implicated in the development of cardiovascular disease. Inflammatory processes can affect blood vessels and influence lipid metabolism.

8. Association with Low HDL Cholesterol: High sugar intake has been linked to lower levels of HDL cholesterol, the "good" cholesterol. HDL cholesterol is essential for transporting cholesterol away from the arteries and back to the liver for excretion.

9. Dietary Sources of Added Sugars: Sugary beverages, processed foods, sweets, and desserts are common sources of added sugars in the diet. Regular consumption of these items can contribute to excessive sugar intake.

10. Complex Carbohydrates vs. Simple Sugars: While complex carbohydrates found in whole grains, fruits, and vegetables contribute essential nutrients and fiber, simple sugars from processed foods can lead to metabolic imbalances and adverse effects on cholesterol.

11. Role of Insulin in Cholesterol Metabolism: Insulin, which is released in response to elevated blood sugar levels, plays a role in lipid metabolism. Dysregulation of insulin due to chronic high sugar intake can influence cholesterol levels.

12. Individual Variability: It's essential to recognize that individual responses to sugar intake vary. Genetic factors, overall diet, lifestyle, and underlying health conditions all play a role in determining how sugars impact cholesterol levels.

13. Guidelines for Added Sugar Intake: Health organizations, including the World Health Organization (WHO) and the American Heart Association (AHA), provide guidelines for recommended daily limits of added sugar intake. Adhering to these guidelines can support overall cardiovascular health.

14. Balancing Macronutrients: Achieving a balanced diet that includes a mix of carbohydrates, proteins, and healthy fats is crucial. This approach, combined with mindful sugar consumption, supports optimal cholesterol levels.

15. Whole Foods Emphasis: Emphasizing whole, unprocessed foods in the diet provides essential nutrients and helps minimize excessive sugar intake. Whole foods contribute to overall health and cardiovascular well-being.

16. Importance of Fiber: Consuming fiber-rich foods, such as fruits, vegetables, and whole grains, helps manage blood sugar levels and supports healthy cholesterol profiles.

17. Regular Health Check-ups: Regular health check-ups, including cholesterol screenings, are essential for monitoring cardiovascular health. These screenings can help detect and address any unfavorable changes in cholesterol levels.

18. Lifestyle Modifications: Incorporating lifestyle modifications, including a balanced diet, regular physical activity, and stress management, can collectively contribute to maintaining healthy cholesterol

Heart-Healthy Recipes and Nutritional Guidelines

Promoting heart health involves embracing a nutrient-rich, balanced diet that supports overall well-being. Here, we delve into heart-healthy recipes and nutritional guidelines, offering a comprehensive approach to nourishing your cardiovascular system:

Nutritional Guidelines for Heart Health

1. Prioritize fruits, vegetables, whole grains, legumes, and nuts. These foods are rich in fiber, antioxidants, and essential nutrients beneficial for heart health.

2. Opt for lean protein sources such as poultry, fish, tofu, beans, and legumes. Limit red meat and processed meats, which can be high in saturated fats.

3. Choose heart-healthy fats like avocados, nuts, seeds, and olive oil. These fats contain monounsaturated and polyunsaturated fats that support cardiovascular health.

4. Prioritize complex carbohydrates found in whole grains, sweet potatoes, and legumes. These carbs provide sustained energy without causing rapid spikes in blood sugar.

5. Reduce intake of foods high in saturated and trans fats. Opt for healthier cooking methods like baking, grilling, or steaming instead of frying.

6. Monitor sodium intake by minimizing processed and packaged foods. Use herbs and spices to flavor meals instead of excessive salt.

7. Incorporate fatty fish like salmon, mackerel, or trout into your diet for omega-3 fatty acids. Alternatively, consider plant-based sources like flaxseeds and chia seeds.

8. If you decide to consume alcohol, do so sparingly. For most adults, moderate drinking is

defined as up to one drink per day for women and up to two drinks per day for men.

9. Increase fiber intake with whole foods like whole grains, fruits, vegetables, and legumes. Fiber supports digestion and helps manage cholesterol levels.

Heart-Healthy Recipes

1. Grilled Salmon with Lemon and Herbs: Marinate salmon fillets in a mixture of lemon juice, olive oil, garlic, and fresh herbs. Grill until cooked through. Serve with a side of quinoa and steamed broccoli.

2. Mediterranean Chickpea Salad: Combine chickpeas, cherry tomatoes, cucumber, red onion, feta cheese, and Kalamata olives. For a cool salad, toss with olive oil, lemon juice, and herbs.

3. Vegetarian Stir-Fry: Stir-fry tofu or tempeh with a colorful array of vegetables like bell peppers, broccoli, and snap peas. Season with ginger, garlic, and a low-sodium soy sauce.

4. Quinoa and Black Bean Bowl: Mix cooked quinoa with black beans, corn, diced tomatoes, avocado, and cilantro. Drizzle with lime juice for a nutrient-packed bowl.

5. Oven-Baked Chicken with Herbs: Coat chicken breasts with a blend of olive oil, rosemary, thyme,

and garlic. Bake until golden brown. Serve with roasted sweet potatoes and green beans.

6. Greek Yogurt Parfait: Layer Greek yogurt with fresh berries, granola, and a drizzle of honey for a delicious and satisfying parfait.

7. Vegetable and Lentil Soup: Simmer lentils with a medley of vegetables like carrots, celery, and spinach. Season with herbs like cumin and coriander for a hearty, heart-healthy soup.

8. Whole Grain Pasta with Pesto and Vegetables: Toss whole grain pasta with homemade pesto, cherry tomatoes, and spinach. Garnish with grated Parmesan for a flavorful pasta dish.

9. Roasted Vegetable Tacos: Roast a variety of vegetables such as bell peppers, zucchini, and onions. Fill whole-grain tortillas with the roasted veggies, black beans, and a sprinkle of cheese.

10. Berry Smoothie with Chia Seeds: Blend mixed berries with Greek yogurt, a banana, and a tablespoon of chia seeds for a nutrient-rich smoothie.

Tips for Heart-Healthy Cooking

1. Choose oils like olive oil, canola oil, or avocado oil for cooking and dressing salads.

2. Minimize the use of processed and packaged foods that often contain hidden salts, sugars, and unhealthy fats.

3. Enhance flavor without excess salt by experimenting with herbs and spices in your cooking.

4. Choose whole grains such as brown rice, quinoa, and whole wheat pasta over refined grains for added fiber and nutrients.

5. Plan your meals ahead of time to ensure a well-balanced and heart-healthy diet. Prep ingredients and consider batch cooking for convenience.

6. Stay informed about nutrition and heart-healthy eating guidelines. Keep updated on new recipes and cooking techniques to make wholesome meals enjoyable.

By incorporating these nutritional guidelines and heart-healthy recipes into your lifestyle, you can actively contribute to maintaining cardiovascular health. Remember, it's always beneficial to consult with healthcare professionals or a registered dietitian for personalized advice based on your specific health needs and goals.

Lifestyle Changes for Improved Cardiovascular Health

Enhancing cardiovascular health involves a comprehensive commitment to lifestyle changes that address various aspects of daily living.

Adopting a heart-healthy lifestyle encompasses dietary choices, physical activity, stress management, and overall well-being. Here's a comprehensive guide to lifestyle changes for improved cardiovascular health:

1. Heart-Healthy Diet

Plant-Based Emphasis: Prioritize a plant-based diet rich in fruits, vegetables, whole grains, legumes, and nuts. These foods provide essential nutrients, fiber, and antioxidants beneficial for heart health.

Lean Proteins: Choose lean protein sources such as fish, poultry, tofu, and legumes. Limit red meat and processed meats, as they can contribute to elevated cholesterol levels.

Healthy Fats: Incorporate heart-healthy fats from sources like olive oil, avocados, nuts, and seeds. These fats support cholesterol balance and overall cardiovascular well-being.

Limit Sodium Intake: Control sodium intake by minimizing processed and packaged foods. Opt for herbs and spices to season meals instead of excessive salt.

2. Regular Physical Activity

Aerobic Exercise: Engage in regular aerobic activities such as brisk walking, jogging, cycling, or swimming. Try to get in at least 150 minutes a week of moderate-to-intense activity.

Strength Training: Include strength training exercises at least two days a week to enhance muscle strength and overall fitness.
Flexibility Exercises: Incorporate flexibility exercises like yoga or stretching to improve joint flexibility and reduce the risk of injuries.
Stay Active Throughout the Day: Break up sedentary periods by incorporating short bouts of activity throughout the day, such as taking stairs or going for short walks.

3. Maintain a Healthy Weight

Balanced Caloric Intake: Achieve and maintain a healthy weight by balancing caloric intake with physical activity. For individualized advice, speak with a qualified dietician or other medical practitioner.
Portion Control: Practice portion control to prevent overeating. Be mindful of serving sizes to avoid excess calorie consumption.

4. Stress Management

Mindfulness Practices: Incorporate mindfulness techniques such as meditation, deep breathing, or yoga to manage stress. These practices can positively impact blood pressure and overall cardiovascular health.
Time Management: Organize and prioritize tasks to reduce feelings of overwhelm. Stress reduction can be enhanced by efficient time management.

5. Adequate Sleep

Consistent Sleep Schedule:Aim for 7-9 hours of quality sleep per night. Establish a consistent sleep schedule to support overall well-being and cardiovascular health.

Sleep Hygiene Practices: Create a conducive sleep environment by minimizing noise, light, and electronic devices before bedtime.

6. Quit Smoking:

Tobacco Cessation: If you smoke, seek support to quit smoking. Smoking is a major risk factor for cardiovascular disease, and quitting has immediate and long-term health benefits.

7. Limit Alcohol Consumption

The key is moderation: If you decide to consume alcohol, do so sparingly. For most adults, moderate drinking is defined as up to one drink per day for women and up to two drinks per day for men.

8. Regular Health Check-ups

Routine Screenings: Schedule regular check-ups with your healthcare provider. Screenings for blood pressure, cholesterol levels, and other cardiovascular risk factors are crucial for early detection and intervention.

9. Social Connections

Supportive Relationships: Cultivate strong social connections and maintain supportive relationships. Positive social interactions contribute to mental well-being, reducing stress and promoting heart health.

10. Hydration

Adequate Water Intake: Stay hydrated with water throughout the day. Proper hydration supports overall health and can contribute to optimal cardiovascular function.

11. Regular Health Education

Stay Informed: Stay informed about heart health through reputable sources. Regularly educate yourself about the latest guidelines and advancements in cardiovascular health.

12. Healthy Cooking and Meal Preparation

Meals Prepared at Home: Make meals at home with whole, fresh ingredients. Cooking at home allows better control over ingredients and portion sizes.
Experiment with Heart-Healthy Recipes: Explore and experiment with heart-healthy recipes that emphasize nutrient-dense foods.

13. Screen Time Management

Digital Detox:** Limit screen time and take breaks from electronic devices. Excessive screen time can contribute to sedentary behavior and disrupt sleep patterns.

14. Financial Wellness

Budgeting and Planning: Financial stress can impact overall well-being. Establish a budget, prioritize financial goals, and seek professional advice if needed.

15. Environmental Considerations

Clean Air: Be mindful of environmental factors that may affect cardiovascular health, such as air pollution. Aim for clean air surroundings and limit your exposure to toxins.

16. Regular Dental Care

Oral Health Connection: Maintain regular dental check-ups. Poor oral health has been linked to cardiovascular disease, emphasizing the importance of dental care.

17. Continuous Learning and Hobbies

Intellectual Stimulation: Engage in continuous learning and pursue hobbies to stimulate the mind. Mental well-being contributes to overall health.

18. Caffeine Moderation

Mindful Caffeine Intake: Limit caffeine intake, especially in the afternoon and evening, to support quality sleep.

19. Healthy Snacking

Nutrient-Rich Snacks: Choose heart-healthy snacks such as fruits, nuts, and yogurt. Avoid excessive consumption of processed snacks high in unhealthy fats and sugars.

20. Community Engagement
Community Activities: Participate in community activities or volunteer work. Social engagement and contributing to the community can enhance mental and emotional well-being.

21. Periodic Reevaluation
Assess and Adjust: Periodically assess your lifestyle choices and make adjustments as needed. As circumstances change, adapting your habits ensures continued cardiovascular well-being.

22. Health Tracker Utilization
Monitoring Health Metrics: Use health trackers or apps to monitor physical activity, sleep patterns, and other health metrics. Tracking progress can motivate and provide valuable insights.

23. Empowerment through Education
Knowledge is Power: Educate yourself about cardiovascular health, risk factors, and preventive measures. Empowerment through knowledge facilitates informed decision-making.

24. Mindful Eating Practices
Conscious Eating:** Practice mindful eating by paying attention to hunger and fullness cues. Enjoy your meals slowly and savor the flavors, fostering a positive relationship with food.

25. Outdoor Activities

Nature Connection: Spend time outdoors engaging in activities like walking, hiking, or gardening. Connecting with nature contributes to both physical and mental well-being.

Adopting these lifestyle changes creates a holistic foundation for improved cardiovascular health. It's essential to approach these changes as long-term commitments, recognizing that small, consistent efforts accumulate to significant benefits over time. As with any health-related adjustments,

CHAPTER SEVEN

Meal Planning and Grocery Shopping Guides

Embarking on a journey toward healthier eating habits involves not just mindful meal planning but also savvy grocery shopping. The synergy between these two aspects forms the foundation of a well-balanced and nutritious lifestyle. In this exploration of Meal Planning and Grocery Shopping Guides, we unravel the secrets to efficient planning, smart ingredient selection, and the art of transforming a shopping cart into a vessel of well-being. Let's dive into the world where thoughtful preparation meets the aisles of wholesome choices, paving the way for a nourishing culinary adventure.

Weekly Meal Plans for Success

Crafting a weekly meal plan is not just a culinary chore; it's a strategic approach to fueling your body with vitality and flavor. Whether your goal is weight management, improved health, or simply savoring delicious meals, a well-thought-out weekly meal plan can be your guiding light. Here's a comprehensive guide to creating and executing successful weekly meal plans:

1. Identify your nutritional goals, whether it's weight loss, muscle gain, or overall well-being. Tailor your meal plan to align with these objectives.

2. Account for dietary preferences, allergies, or restrictions. A flexible meal plan accommodates your unique needs and ensures enjoyment.

3. Include a mix of macronutrients (carbohydrates, proteins, and fats) and micronutrients (vitamins and minerals) in each meal for comprehensive nutrition.

4. Map out your week with a calendar. Allocate specific meals for each day, considering your schedule and potential time constraints.

5. Embrace variety to prevent monotony. Rotate proteins, grains, vegetables, and flavors to keep your taste buds engaged.

6. Optimize time with batch cooking and meal prep. Prepare staples like grains, proteins, and sauces in advance for quicker assembly during the week.

7. Don't forget hydration. Plan for an adequate intake of water throughout the day, and consider incorporating herbal teas or infused water for variety.

8. Stay flexible. Life is dynamic, and plans may change. Be adaptable and have contingency options for busy days or unexpected events.

9. Create a detailed grocery list based on your meal plan. To make shopping easier, arrange it according to sections.

10. Stick to your grocery list and avoid impulse buys. Shop with purpose, focusing on nutrient-dense foods.

11. Embrace seasonal and local produce. They are often fresher, more flavorful, and support sustainability.

12. Allow for occasional treats. A well-balanced meal plan accommodates indulgences, promoting a sustainable and enjoyable approach to eating.

13. Periodically review your meal plan. Evaluate what went well and what needs to be improved. Adjust the plan based on your evolving preferences and goals.

14. If planning for a family, consider everyone's preferences. Engage family members in the process to ensure collective satisfaction.

15. Infuse creativity into your plan. Experiment with new recipes and cuisines to keep your culinary journey exciting.

16. Be attuned to how your body responds to different foods. Listen to hunger and fullness cues, fostering a mindful eating practice.

By embracing the art of weekly meal planning, you not only nourish your body but also cultivate a positive and sustainable relationship with food. It's a journey where every meal becomes a step toward your well-being, and each plan sets the stage for a week of culinary triumphs.

Smart Grocery Shopping

Navigating the aisles with intentionality can transform your grocery shopping experience into a journey toward a sugar-free lifestyle. Whether you're aiming to manage your weight, regulate blood sugar, or enhance overall well-being, choosing sugar-free ingredients is a pivotal step. Here's a comprehensive guide to smart grocery shopping, empowering you to select ingredients that align with a sugar-free lifestyle:

1. Prioritize Whole Foods
    - Embrace the periphery of the grocery store, where fresh produce, lean proteins, and whole grains are often located. Whole foods are naturally lower in added sugars.

2. Read Nutrition Labels
    - Scrutinize nutrition labels for hidden sugars. Ingredients like high-fructose corn syrup, sucrose, and other syrups may be disguised under different names.

3. Identify Natural Sugars
    - Distinguish between natural sugars present in fruits and dairy versus added sugars. Whole fruits and unsweetened dairy can be part of a balanced diet.

4. Choose Low-Glycemic Options
    - Opt for foods with a low glycemic index to help manage blood sugar levels. Legumes, whole grains, and non-starchy veggies are a few of these.

5. Explore Sugar Alternatives
   - Consider sugar alternatives like stevia, erythritol, or monk fruit for sweetening without the added sugars. Ensure they are suitable for your dietary preferences and health goals.

6. Minimize Processed Foods
   - Processed foods often harbor hidden sugars. Minimize their presence in your cart, focusing instead on fresh, whole ingredients.

7. Choose Whole Grains
   - When selecting grains, opt for whole grains like quinoa, brown rice, and oats. These provide complex carbohydrates without the rapid sugar spikes.

8. Mindful Protein Selection
   - Check labels on protein sources, such as yogurt and packaged meats. Choose options without added sugars or opt for plain varieties and add your own flavorings.

9. Select Unsweetened Beverages
   - Choose unsweetened beverages like water, herbal teas, or black coffee. Sugary drinks contribute significantly to added sugar intake.

10. Stock Up on Fresh Produce
   - Put a rainbow of fresh fruits and veggies in your shopping. These nutrient-rich options are naturally low in added sugars.

11. Lean Protein Choices

- Choose lean protein sources like poultry, fish, tofu, and legumes. Minimize processed and breaded options, as they may contain added sugars.

12. Check Condiment Labels

- Review labels on condiments, sauces, and dressings. Opt for options with little to no added sugars or explore making your own at home.

13. Dairy without Added Sugars

- Select dairy products without added sugars. Plain yogurt, unsweetened almond milk, and natural cheeses are sugar-free alternatives.

14. Frozen Vegetables and Fruits

- Utilize frozen vegetables and fruits without added sugars. They are convenient, retain nutritional value, and offer versatility in meal preparation.

15. Mindful Snacking Choices

- Choose snacks wisely. Nuts, seeds, and fresh fruits make excellent sugar-free snacks, providing both energy and nutrients.

16. Smart Bakery Choices

- If purchasing bakery items, opt for whole-grain, sugar-free options or explore baking at home using sugar alternatives.

17. Conduct Price and Unit Comparisons

- Consider price and unit comparisons to make informed choices. Sometimes, healthier options can be cost-effective when considering long-term health benefits.

18. Explore Ethnic Foods

- Explore ethnic foods that traditionally use fewer added sugars. Mediterranean, Asian, and Latin cuisines often feature flavorful dishes without excessive sweetness.

19. Plan Meals in Advance

- Plan your meals in advance to streamline grocery shopping. Having a clear list helps you resist impulse purchases that may be high in added sugars.

20. Educate Yourself on Food Labels

- Familiarize yourself with common terms used on food labels, such as "no added sugars," "unsweetened," or "sugar-free."

21. Be Wary of "Low-Fat" Products

- Some low-fat products compensate for taste by adding sugars. Read labels carefully and prioritize nutrient-dense options.

22. Dried Fruits in Moderation
   - If choosing dried fruits, do so in moderation. While nutritious, they can be concentrated sources of natural sugars.

23. Avoid Sugary Cereals
   - Opt for whole-grain, low-sugar cereals. Many breakfast cereals contain high amounts of added sugars.

24. DIY Salad Dressings
   - Create homemade salad dressings using olive oil, vinegar, and herbs. This ensures you control the ingredients and avoid unnecessary sugars.

25. Check Sugar Content in Baby Foods
   - If shopping for baby foods, check labels for added sugars. Choose options with minimal or no added sugars to instill healthy eating habits early.

26. Utilize Online Resources
   - Leverage online resources and apps that provide information on the sugar content of various foods. Stay informed to make educated choices.

By applying these strategies, your grocery shopping endeavors become a purposeful and health-conscious activity. The key lies in informed choices, label literacy, and a commitment to nourishing your body with wholesome, sugar-free ingredients. Transform your cart into a vehicle of well-being and embark on a journey toward a healthier, sugar-conscious lifestyle.

CHAPTER EIGHT

A sample 7-day meal plan

Day 1

Breakfast:
- Scrambled Eggs with Spinach and Tomatoes
- Whole Grain Toast

Lunch:
- Grilled Chicken Salad with Mixed Greens, Cucumbers, and Avocado
- Olive Oil and Lemon Dressing

Dinner:
- Baked Salmon with Lemon and Dill
- Quinoa Pilaf
- Steamed Broccoli

Day 2

Breakfast:
- Greek Yogurt Parfait with Berries and Almonds

Lunch:
- Lentil and Vegetable Soup
- Whole Grain Crackers

Dinner:
- Turkey and Vegetable Stir-Fry
- Cauliflower Rice

Day 3

Breakfast:
- Chia Seed Pudding with Unsweetened Almond Milk and Fresh Berries

Lunch:
- Quinoa Salad with Chickpeas, Cherry Tomatoes, and Feta Cheese
- Lemon Vinaigrette

Dinner:
- Grilled Shrimp Skewers
- Roasted Sweet Potatoes
- Asparagus Spears

Day 4

Breakfast:
- Bell peppers, mushrooms, and feta cheese in an omelette

Lunch:
- Tuna Salad Lettuce Wraps
- Sliced Cucumber on the side

Dinner:
- Baked Chicken Breast with Herbs
- Brown Rice
- Steamed Green Beans

Day 5

Breakfast:

- Avocado and Tomato on Whole Grain Toast

Lunch:
- Quinoa and Black Bean Bowl with Salsa
- Sliced Avocado

Dinner:
- Grilled Cod with Garlic and Herb Marinade
- Quinoa Salad with Cucumber and Mint

Day 6

Breakfast:
- Protein powder, spinach, banana, and unsweetened almond milk blended into a smoothie.

Lunch:
- Turkey Lettuce Wraps with Hummus
- Carrot Sticks

Dinner:
- Baked Eggplant Parmesan with Marinara Sauce
- Zucchini Noodles

Day 7

Breakfast:
- Cottage Cheese with Sliced Peaches

Lunch:
- Chicken and Vegetable Skewers
- Brown Rice

Dinner
- Grilled Steak with Chimichurri Sauce
- Roasted Brussels Sprouts

Feel free to adapt these recipes based on your preferences and dietary needs. Keep in mind to stay hydrated throughout the day and pay attention to your body's signals of hunger and fullness. Enjoy your journey into a sugar-free lifestyle!

WHO and AHA guidelines for recommended daily limits of added sugar intake

Both the World Health Organization (WHO) and the American Heart Association (AHA) provide guidelines for recommended daily limits of added sugar intake. These guidelines aim to help individuals make informed dietary choices and reduce the risk of health issues associated with excessive sugar consumption.

World Health Organization (WHO)

The WHO recommends that both adults and children limit their intake of free sugars. Free sugars include sugars added to foods and beverages by the manufacturer, cook, or consumer, plus sugars naturally present in honey, syrups, and fruit juices.

WHO Guidelines
1. **Adults and Children**
Free sugar intake should be less than 10% of total daily energy intake.
A further reduction to below 5% of total daily energy intake is encouraged for additional health benefits.

2. **Children Under 2 Years Old**
It is recommended to avoid the use of free sugars in the diet of children under 2 years.

3. **Practical Tips**
Consume a variety of foods rich in whole fruits, vegetables, whole grains, and nuts.
Limit the intake of sugary snacks and beverages, including sodas and processed foods.

American Heart Association (AHA)

The AHA provides specific recommendations for added sugar intake to promote heart health. These guidelines are based on the concept of discretionary calorie allowance, which accounts for the total number of calories an individual can consume while meeting their nutritional needs.

AHA Guidelines
1. **Adult Men**
Limit daily added sugar intake to no more than 9 teaspoons (36 grams) or 150 calories.

2. **Adult Women**
Limit daily added sugar intake to no more than 6 teaspoons (25 grams) or 100 calories.

3. **Children (2–18 years old)**
 Limit daily added sugar intake to no more than 6 teaspoons (25 grams) or 100 calories.

4. **Practical Tips**
Read food labels to identify sources of added sugars.
Choose foods and beverages with little or no added sugars.
Limit the consumption of sugary drinks and snacks.

Both the WHO and AHA emphasize the importance of reducing added sugar intake to support overall health, reduce the risk of obesity, and prevent chronic diseases such as cardiovascular diseases and type 2 diabetes. Individuals are encouraged to be mindful of their sugar intake and make informed choices for a balanced and healthful diet.

CONCLUSION

As we bid farewell to the journey through "No Sugar Diet for Beginners," the echoes of transformative change linger in the air. This comprehensive guide, penned with a commitment to your well-being, has illuminated the path toward a sugar-free lifestyle—one laden with wholesome choices, nourishing recipes, and strategic insights into weight management, diabetes, and cholesterol control.

In our exploration of the impact of sugar on health, we uncovered the intricate connections between dietary choices and overall well-being. From unraveling the mysteries of blood sugar spikes to understanding the profound effects on mental health and chronic diseases, each revelation has served as a beacon, guiding us away from the pitfalls of excess sugar consumption.

The heart of this journey lies in the practical application of knowledge. From defining added sugars versus natural sugars to mastering the art of reading labels and overcoming sugar cravings, you've been equipped with the tools needed to navigate the modern food landscape consciously.
The recipes generously shared throughout these pages are not mere culinary suggestions but invitations to savor a symphony of flavors without the burden of excessive sugars. From energizing breakfast delights to satisfying dinner creations and

guilt-free snacks, each recipe encapsulates the essence of a sugar-free lifestyle—one that delights the palate and nurtures the body.

Understanding the link between sugar and weight gain has empowered you to make informed choices, providing strategies that prioritize health without sacrificing flavor. We explored the delicate balance required for diabetes management through dietary choices, offering practical tips for daily well-being.

The journey reached its crescendo with insights into naturally lowering cholesterol, fortifying your heart's health through heart-friendly recipes and embracing lifestyle changes for improved cardiovascular well-being.

As you turn the last page, remember that the conclusion of this book is not an end but a commencement—a commencement of a healthier tomorrow. The commitment you've made to a sugar-free lifestyle is a gift to your future self, an investment in vitality, and an affirmation of the vibrant, well-balanced life you deserve.

So, as you embark on the sweet journey ahead, may it be adorned with the sweetness of fruits, the richness of wholesome meals, and the joy of a healthier, more energetic you. Farewell to sugary habits, and here's to embracing a future where your health is the sweetest reward.